# Shared Governance

## A Practical Approach to Reshaping
## Professional Nursing Practice

Diana Swihart, PhD, DMin, MSN, CS, APRN,BC

Foreword by *Tim Porter-O'Grady, EdD, APRN, FAAN*

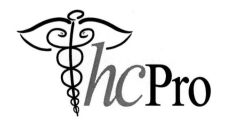

*Shared Governance: A Practical Approach to Reshaping Professional Nursing Practice* is published by HCPro, Inc.

Diana Swihart, PhD, DMin, MSN, CS, APRN,BC, Author
Jamie Gisonde, Senior Managing Editor
Emily Sheahan, Group Publisher
Patrick Campagnone, Cover Designer
Shane Katz, Graphic Artist
Mike Michaud, Bookbuilder
Jean St. Pierre, Director of Operations
Darren Kelly, Production Coordinator
Lauren Rubenzahl, Copyeditor

Advice given is general. Readers should consult professional counsel for specific legal, ethical, or clinical questions. Arrangements can be made for quantity discounts. For more information, contact

HCPro, Inc.
P.O. Box 1168
Marblehead, MA 01945
Telephone: 800/650-6787 or 781/639-1872
Fax: 781/639-2982
E-mail: *customerservice@hcpro.com*

**Visit HCPro, Inc., at its World Wide Web sites: *www.hcpro.com* and *www.hcmarketplace.com***

Rev. 09/2007
21469

# Contents

# About the author

## Diana Swihart, PhD, DMin, MSN, CS, APRN,BC

**Diana Swihart, PhD, DMin, MSN, CS, APRN,BC,** a clinical nurse specialist in nursing education at the Bay Pines (FL) VA Healthcare System, has a diverse background that includes many professional nursing arenas, theology, ministry, ancient Near Eastern studies, and archaeology. She is a member of the editorial advisory board for Advance for Nurses, Florida edition, and has published and spoken on numerous topics related to nursing, shared governance, competency assessment, education, and staff development, both locally and nationally. She has served as an ANCC Magnet Recognition Program® appraiser and is currently the treasurer for the National Nursing Staff Development Organization (NNSDO). Her training and experiences, including those in academic and staff development education, give her a broad and balanced perspective of nursing that influences and colors all that she does as she challenges and encourages others through professional nurse development in professional practice environments of care.

# About the contributors

## Katherine Riley, BSN, RN, CNA,BC

*Southwestern Vermont Medical Center, Bennington, an ANCC Magnet Recognition Program®
organization since 2002*

**Katherine Riley, BSN, RN, CNA,BC** is the ANCC Magnet Recognition Program® (MRP)
coordinator and assistant vice president of operations at Southwestern Vermont Medical
Center (SVMC) in Bennington. Riley helped develop SVMC's clinical advancement programs for nursing and imaging services, led the implementation of a shared governance
model of professional practice across all clinical disciplines, and initiated a staff-supported
salary model for women's and children's services—all of which were key ingredients to the
hospital's designation. In 2001, Riley led SVMC's MRP first application process, and she
continues to oversee the development of the hospital's MRP culture. SVMC successfully
earned redesignation earlier this year.

## Polly H. Willis, MSN, RN

*Saint Joseph's Hospital, Atlanta, an ANCC Magnet Recognition Program® organization since 1995*

**Polly H. Willis, MSN, RN,** has been a nurse for more than 30 years, spending much of
her career at Saint Joseph's Hospital. She has provided direct patient care in med-surg and
critical care services. In 1990, she became the quality improvement coordinator for Saint
Joseph's and led the implementation of the department of patient care management. In her
role as director of this department, she oversaw the functions of case management, utilization review, discharge planning, social services, infection control, and quality improvement.
In 1999, Willis became a cardiology case manager at Saint Joseph's and served as the primary author of the institution's written documentation for redesignation, which it achieved
in 2000. In 2001, she became the nursing director of two med-surg telemetry units, acute
dialysis services at Saint Joseph's, and a 24-bed med-surg critical care unit. In 2002, Willis
was named the MRP coordinator and the director of Saint Joseph's Stroke Center. She was
the primary author of the MRP documentation completed successfully for redesignation
2004. Willis has also provided many consultations and presentations through Saint Joseph's
Kenneth E. Thomas Center for Nursing Excellence on designation and shared governance.

# Acknowledgements

Every work, regardless of scope and size, is completed only with the help and inspiration of others. My sincere thanks go to my beloved husband for his support and encouragement, and for his unwavering belief in me. I also want to thank my devoted son, who lent his own writing skills and gifts to the reading and early critiquing of the manuscript, helping me write in a way that would be more comfortable and interesting for readers.

I would also like to acknowledge those speakers and teachers who have contributed their ideas and thoughts through countless classes, seminars, and lectures that I have attended over the years. I write from their influence and want to recognize their contributions, although their names are too numerous to list.

Finally, I would like to salute Dr. Tim Porter-O'Grady, whose work first drew me to the study of shared governance. After studying more than 176 of his articles, videos, and books, my ideas and writing most strongly reflect his influence. For this reason, I am particularly pleased that Dr. Porter-O'Grady has written the foreword for what I hope to be a valuable addition to your own journey in helping reshape professional nursing practice for this generation and the next.

*Diana Swihart*

Diana Swihart

# Foreword

The concept of shared governance is not new. Engaging and empowering people, the centerpiece of shared governance, has been associated with good management for some 60 years. It seems to many that such concepts are new and innovative simply because so few leaders actually implement these concepts into the exercise of their own management. The prevailing model for management has historically been one that represents parent-child relationships, since it is the predominant model of leadership that most people can identify in the absence of real leadership education.

In nursing, much of management represents a parental and maternal influence that extends into the staff management interaction at every level of nursing practice. From the orientation program to policy, procedure, protocols, and practices, the nurse is constantly reminded of how much her or his life is scripted and controlled by external parameters and directives. It is no wonder that, given enough time, most nurses lose interest in controlling their own practice and influencing the practice lives of others. Ultimately, a nurse's locus of control becomes so narrow that he or she ceases to do anything but the most functional and routine activities and quickly becomes addicted to the predictable and ritualistic functional activities of nursing.

It is a challenge to get nurses out of their rut and fully engage them in their practice lives. Even when it is clearly in the best interest of the nurse to become more fully involved, the vagaries of work, the demands of patient care, and any other excuse becomes the barrier to fully engaging with those things that are necessary to advance and change practice. The leaders, for their part, have created such a vertical orientation and relationship that staff ultimately feel as though anything significant, important, or valuable can only be done by managers or by management mandate. They feel that any effort on the part of the staff infringes on their time and therefore is not legitimate.

Shared governance reflects a completely different mental model for relationship and for leadership. It recognizes that nursing is a profession and requires the professional frame for how it is structured and does its business. In fact, shared governance is predominantly about building a particular infrastructure or framework for the "professionalization" of nursing. It re-orients the decision-making construct to require a broader distribution of decisions across the profession and allocates decisions based on accountability and role expectations. This re-configuration of the nursing organization is intended to define staff-based decisions, accountability, roles, and ownership of staff in those activities that directly affect the nurse's life and practice.

Success with shared governance requires a powerful reorientation of the organization. It requires leadership to understand that a significant re-tooling of leadership capacity and skill is required to successfully implement shared governance and sustain it as a way of life in the professional organization. Implementing shared governance means retraining managers, engaging staff, reallocating accountability, and building a truly staff-driven model of decision and action. Because behavior cannot be changed or sustained without a supporting infrastructure, it means redesigning and structuring the organization to eliminate rewards for passive behavior and enumerating and inculcating rewards for engagement within the very fabric of the organization.

Staff-driven decision-making is a strong indicator of excellence. It is no surprise that ANCC Magnet Recognition® has numerous Forces of Magnetism that reflect the values and system of shared governance and staff-based accountability. Also, the work is not easy, and it cannot be done overnight. It means building an entire new culture that clearly and unambiguously reflects the characteristics of a truly professional organization. From the highest levels of organizational leadership to the patient relationship, there must be strong evidence of practice driving the organization's work. In all professions, power is grounded in practice. Excellence in practice can only be obtained and sustained if the practitioners hold and exercise the power that only practice can drive in achieving excellence and satisfaction. Without it, the power to influence, change, challenge, and "push the walls" toward innovation and creativity is simply vacated, and others end up playing that role, whether their doing so is legitimate or not.

Sharon Finnigan and I wrote the first definitive book on shared governance in 1985. Although we and others have continued to add to that body of knowledge over the years, no substantial foundational text on implementing the basics of an effective shared governance system has been forthcoming since that time, until this current work. Here, the author has clearly enumerated the foundations of shared governance and the practical elements necessary to construct a shared governance structure and to make it successful. This is perhaps one of the clearest explications of the principles, design, and processes associated with a viable and successful shared governance model that exists in the literature today.

If the reader carefully works through this text and thoughtfully reasons and applies the principles set out herein, he or she can advance the opportunity to create a successful approach to shared governance. Each stage of development, every design element, components of the decision process, and evaluation of effectiveness outlined here provides the tools necessary to make implementation successful. Although the work will be focused and sometimes difficult, the rewards have proven to be substantial to those who have been willing to risk the effort and initiate the dynamic of creating a truly professional nursing organization. There is no greater indicator of a viable and sustainable potential for nursing and nurses—as well as those we serve—than a fully empowered and engaged profession that creates the foundations and conditions for excellence for the foreseeable future.

Tim Porter-O'Grady

# Chapter 1

# Introduction: The concept behind shared governance

## Learning objectives

After reading this chapter, the participant should be able to do the following:

- Define the four primary principles of shared governance: partnership, equity, accountability, and ownership.
- Compare two professional nursing practice models.
- Describe the role of relational partnerships in shared governance.

*"Nursing is the protection, promotion, and optimization of health and abilities, prevention of illness and injury, alleviation of suffering through the diagnosis and treatment of human response, and advocacy in the care of individuals, families, communities, and populations."* —American Nurses Association (2003)

The increasingly critical shortage of professional nurses is a dangerous theme in healthcare. In response to it, more and more institutions are turning to shared governance—a concept introduced into healthcare organizations in the 1970s—as an evidence-based method to curb the shortage's damaging effects (e.g., negative patient outcomes, high cost of agency staff, and RN sign-on bonuses). This book takes some of the guesswork out of the various structures and processes behind shared governance and provides strategies, case examples, and best practices to make the daily operations of shared governance meaningful and successful. It also explores the relationship between shared governance and the ANCC Magnet Recognition Program® by outlining the program's expectations for shared governance practices.

## What is shared governance?

*"Before it can be solved, a problem must be clearly defined."*
—William Feather

In its simplest form, shared governance is shared decision-making based on the principles of partnership, equity, accountability, and ownership at the point of service. This management process model empowers all members of the healthcare workforce to have a voice in decision-making, thus encouraging diverse and creative input that will help advance the business and healthcare missions of the organization. In essence, it makes every employee feel like he or she is "part manager" with a personal stake in the success of the organization. This feeling leads to

- longevity of employment
- increased employee satisfaction
- better safety and healthcare
- greater patient satisfaction
- shorter lengths of stay

Those who are happy in their jobs take greater ownership of their decisions and are more vested in patient outcomes. Therefore, employees, patients, the organization, and the surrounding communities benefit from shared governance.

## Four principles of shared governance

If shared governance is to allow for cost-effective service delivery and nurse empowerment, decision-making must be shared at point of service—which means that the management structure must be decentralized. To make that happen, employee partnership, equity, accountability, and ownership must occur at the point of service (e.g., on the patient care units). At least 90% of the decisions need to be made there. Indeed, in matters of practice, quality, and competence, the locus of control in the professional practice environment must shift to practitioners. Only 10% of the unit-level decisions should belong to management (Porter-O'Grady and Hinshaw 2005).

- *Partnership*—links healthcare providers and patients along all points in the system; a collaborative relationship among all stakeholders and nursing required for professional empowerment. Partnership is essential to building relationships, involves all staff members in decisions and processes, implies that each member has a key role in fulfilling the mission and purpose of the organization, and is critical to the healthcare system's effectiveness (Porter-O'Grady and Hinshaw 2005; Batson 2004).

- *Equity*—the best method for integrating staff roles and relationships into structures and processes to achieve positive patient outcomes. Equity maintains a focus on services, patients, and staff; is the foundation and measure of value; and says that no one role is more important than any other. Although equity does not equal equality in terms of scope of practice, knowledge, authority, or responsibility, it does mean that each team member is essential to providing safe and effective care (Porter-O'Grady and Hinshaw 2005; Batson 2004; Porter-O'Grady, Hawkins, and Parker 1997).

- *Accountability*—a willingness to invest in decision-making and express ownership in those decisions. Accountability is the core of shared governance. It is often used interchangeably with *responsibility* and allows for evaluation of role performance (see Figure 1.1 for characteristics of accountability and responsibility). It supports partnerships and is secured as staff produce positive outcomes (Porter-O'Grady and Hinshaw 2005; Batson 2004).

## Figure 1.1: Characteristics of accountability and responsibility

| Accountability | Responsibility |
|---|---|
| • Defined by outcomes | • Defined by functions |
| • Self-described | • Delegated |
| • Embedded in roles | • Specific tasks/routines dictated |
| • Dependent on partnerships | • Isolative |
| • Shares evaluation | • Supervisor evaluation |
| • Contributions-driven value | • Tasks-driven value |

*Adapted from T. Porter-O'Grady and K. S. Hinshaw 2005.*

- *Ownership*—recognition and acceptance of the importance of everyone's work and of the fact that an organization's success is bound to how well individual staff members perform their jobs. To enable all team members to participate, ownership designates where work is done and by whom. It requires all staff members to commit to contributing something, to own what they contribute, and to participate in devising purposes for the work (Porter-O'Grady and Hinshaw 2005; Batson 2004; Koloroutis 2004; Page 2004). Shared governance activities may include participatory scheduling, joint staffing decisions, and/or shared unit responsibilities (e.g., every RN is trained to be "in charge" of his or her unit or area and shares that role with other professional team members, perhaps on a rotating schedule) to achieve the best patient care outcomes.

The old centralized management structures for command and control are ineffective for today's healthcare market. They frequently inhibit effective change and growth within the organization and limit future market possibilities in recruitment and retention of qualified nurses. Summative, hierarchical decision-making creates barriers to employee autonomy and empowerment and can undermine service and quality of care. Today's patients are no longer satisfied with directive care. They, too, want partnership, equity, accountability, and mutual ownership in their healthcare decisions and those of their family members.

## History and development of shared governance

The concept of shared governance, or shared decision-making, is not new. Philosophy, education, religion, politics, business and management, and healthcare have all benefited from various shared governance process models implemented in many diverse and creative ways across generations and cultures. For example:

- By the 1950s, shared governance had found its way into the business and management literature (O'May and Buchan 1999; Laschinger 1996; Peters 1991; Walton 1986; Peters and Waterman 1982). Organizations began to design more decentralized, interpersonal structures and relationships among their leaders and employees. They emphasized making decisions from the point of service outward instead of from the organization downward.

- In the late 1970s and early 1980s, shared governance formally found its way into the healthcare and nursing arenas, growing out of nurses' dissatisfaction with the institutions in which they practiced (O'May and Buchan 1999; Porter-O'Grady 1995; McDonagh et al 1989; Cleland 1978). Nurses started to use it as a form of participative management through using self-managed work teams.

The professional practice environment of nursing care has shifted dramatically over the past generation (AONE 2000; AACN 2002). Rapid advances are occurring in

- biotechnology and cyberscience
- disease prevention, patient safety, and management
- relationship-based care
- patients' roles in their healthcare (i.e., they are active partners, not just passive recipients)

Economic constraints related to service reimbursement and corporatism have forced healthcare systems to save money by

- downsizing the professional workforce
- changing staffing mixes

- restructuring/reorganizing services
- reducing support services for patient care
- moving patients more rapidly to alternative care settings or discharge

Poor collaboration and ineffective communication among healthcare providers can result in devastating medical errors. The struggle to provide quality care in the highly stressful—and sometimes highly charged—work environment today has resulted in limited success in recruitment and retention of qualified nurses nationwide (Kohn, Corrigan and Donaldson 1999; AACN 2002; Weinberg 2003).

## Shared governance and professional nursing practice models

As economic realities shift and change, so does nursing practice. Tim Porter-O'Grady (1987) observed, "Reorganization in health care institutions is currently the rule rather than the exception. All health care participants are attempting to strategically position themselves in the marketplace. What do these changes mean for nursing? How can nursing best respond?" (p. 281). It is an even greater challenge today to develop an effective professional nursing practice model for an economically constrained healthcare system to achieve positive outcomes, build workplace advocacy, and provide needed resources and support to improve recruitment and retention of a shrinking nurse workforce.

Anthony (2004) describes some of the nursing models that have evolved to provide structure and context for care delivery:

- Those based on patient assignment (i.e., team nursing)
- Accountability systems (i.e., primary care nursing)
- Managed care (i.e., case management)
- Shared governance, based on professional autonomy and participatory, or shared, decision-making (i.e., relationship-based care)

Koloroutis (2004) presents the integrated work of nurse leaders, researchers, and authors who have worked with a global community of healthcare organizations over the past 25 years. The result is relationship-based care (RBC), a nursing model that lends itself well to shared governance in today's complex healthcare systems (see Figure 1.2 for self governance vs. shared governance).

In the RBC model, nursing services are provided through relationships in a caring and healing environment that embodies the concepts of partnership, equity, accountability, and ownership.

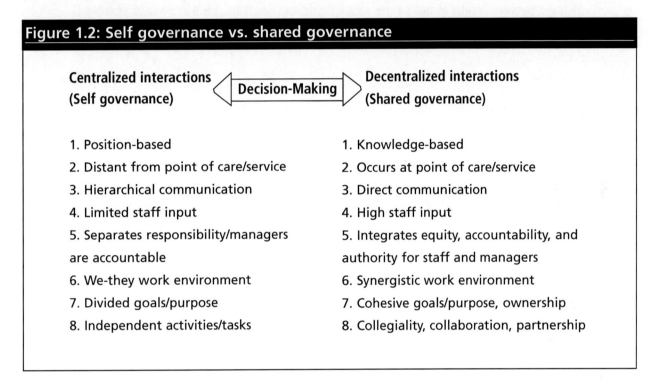

Figure 1.2: Self governance vs. shared governance

Centralized interactions (Self governance)  —  Decision-Making  —  Decentralized interactions (Shared governance)

| Centralized interactions (Self governance) | Decentralized interactions (Shared governance) |
| --- | --- |
| 1. Position-based | 1. Knowledge-based |
| 2. Distant from point of care/service | 2. Occurs at point of care/service |
| 3. Hierarchical communication | 3. Direct communication |
| 4. Limited staff input | 4. High staff input |
| 5. Separates responsibility/managers are accountable | 5. Integrates equity, accountability, and authority for staff and managers |
| 6. We-they work environment | 6. Synergistic work environment |
| 7. Divided goals/purpose | 7. Cohesive goals/purpose, ownership |
| 8. Independent activities/tasks | 8. Collegiality, collaboration, partnership |

Shared decision-making works best in a decentralized organizational structure where those at the point of service make their own decisions and determine whether they are appropriate. "When staff members are clear about their roles, responsibilities, authority, and accountability, they have greater confidence in their own judgments and are more willing to take ownership for decision making at the point of care" (Koloroutis 2004). Decentralized decision-making is most successful when *responsibility, authority, and accountability* (R+A+A) are clearly delineated and assigned (Wright 2002).

- *Responsibility:* the clear and specific allocation of duties to achieve desired results. Assignment of responsibility is a two-way process: It is visibly given and visibly accepted. This acceptance is the essence of responsibility. Note, however, that individuals cannot accept responsibility without a level of authority.

- *Authority:* the right to act and make decisions in the areas where one is given and accepts responsibility. When people are asked to share in the work, they must know their level of authority with regard to that work. Levels of authority determine a person's right to act in the areas he or she is given. There are four levels of authority (Wright 2002):

  1. *Data gathering*—"Get information, bring it back to me, and I will decide what to do with it." Example, *Please go down and see whether Mr. Jones has a headache. Then come back and tell me what he says.*

  2. **Data gathering + recommendations**—"Get the information (collect the data), look at the situation and make some recommendations, and I will pick from one of those recommendations what we will do next. I still decide." Example, *Please go down and see whether Mr. Jones has a headache. Then come back and tell me what you would recommend that I give him.*

  3. **Data gathering + recommendations [pause] + act**—"Get the information (collect the data), look at the situation, make some recommendations, and pick one that you will do. But before you carry it out, I want you to stop (pause) and check with me before you do it." The pause is not necessarily for approval. It is more of a double check, to make sure that everything was considered before proceeding. Example, *Please go down and see whether Mr. Jones has a headache. Then come back and tell me what you would recommend for him; then take care of him for me.*

  4. **Act and inform/update**—"Do what needs to be done and tell me what happened or update me later." There is no pause before the action. Example, *Please take care of Mr. Jones for me.*

- *Accountability*: begins when one reviews and reflects upon his or her own actions and decisions, and culminates with a personal assessment that helps determine the best actions to take in the future.

For example, in shared governance, a nurse manager is accountable for patient care delivery in his or her area of responsibility. The manager does not do all of the tasks but does provide the resources that staff nurses need and ensures that patient care delivery is effective. In that patient care area, the nurse manager/ leader is accountable for setting the direction, looking at past decisions, and evaluating outcomes. Bedside nurses are accountable for the overall care outcomes of assigned groups of patients for the time period they are there and for overseeing the big picture; however, other people (dieticians, therapists, pharmacists, laboratory technicians, and other healthcare providers) share in the responsibility for the subsequent tasks in meeting patients' needs.

Although definitions, models, structures, and principles of shared governance (or *collaborative governance, participatory governance, shared or participatory leadership, staff empowerment,* or *clinical governance*) vary, the outcomes are consistent. The evidence suggests that shared governance processes result in the following:

- Increased nurse satisfaction with shared decision-making, related to increased responsibility that is combined with appropriate authority and accountability
- Increased professional autonomy, as well as higher staff and nurse manager retention
- Greater patient and staff satisfaction
- Improved patient care outcomes
- Better financial states due to cost savings/cost reductions

## Shared governance and relational partnerships

*"The best [leader] is the one who has sense enough to pick good [people] to do what he/she wants done, and self-restraint enough to keep from meddling with them while they do it."* —Theodore Roosevelt

Professional nurses long ago identified shared governance as a key indicator of excellence in nursing practice (McDonagh et al. 1989; Metcalf and Tate 1995; Porter-O'Grady 1987, 2001, 2005). Porter-O'Grady (2001) described shared governance as a process model that provides a structure for organizing nursing work within organizational settings. It empowers nurses to express and manage their practice with a greater degree of professional autonomy. Personal and professional accountability are respected and supported within the organization. In addition, leadership support for point-of-care nurses enables them to maintain quality nursing practice, job satisfaction, and financial viability when partnership, equity, accountability, and ownership are in place (Page 2004; Anthony 2004; Koloroutis 2004; Porter-O'Grady 2003a, 2003b; Green and Jordan 2002).

Today's transformational relationship-based healthcare, which is driven by technology, creates a new paradigm with different goals and objectives in an organizational learning environment. Leaders, administrators, and employees are learning and implementing new ways of providing care, new technologies, and new ways of thinking and working. In the process, they recognize more and more that the nurse at the point of service is key to organizational success.

Nurses and managers must be prepared for new roles, new relationships, and new ways of managing. Shared governance is about moving from a traditional hierarchical model to a relational partnership model of nursing practice (see Figure 1.3).

## Figure 1.3: Hierarchy vs. relational partnership

| From HIERARCHY | to → | RELATIONAL PARTNERSHIP |
| --- | --- | --- |

**From HIERARCHY** → to → **RELATIONAL PARTNERSHIP**

- Independence
- Hierarchical relationship
- Parallel functioning
- Medical plan
- Resisting change
- Competing
- Indirect communication

- Interdependence
- Collegial relationship
- Team functioning
- Patient's plan
- Leading change
- Partnering
- Direct communication

Successful relational partnerships in collaborative practice require understanding the roles of each partner. If the partners are not aware of what each brings to that relationship, they will have considerable problems collaborating, acting responsibly, and being accountable for decisions and care. Therefore, relational partnerships can be a complex and challenging framework for the shared governance professional nursing practice model (Porter-O'Grady and Hinshaw 2005; Green and Jordan 2004; Koloroutis 2004; Porter-O'Grady 2002).

The key provider at point of service—the staff nurse—moves from the bottom to the center of the organization. Nurses are the primary employees who do the work and connect the organization to the recipient of its service. An entirely different sense and set of variables now affect the design of the organization—the only one who matters in a service-based organization is the one who provides its service. All other roles become servant to that role. In this way, the paradigm shifts to a relationship-based, staff-centered, patient-focused professional nursing practice model of care in which nurse managers or supervisors assume the role of *servant leaders* managing resources and outcomes (Nightingale 1992).

When managers become *servant leaders*, they function differently in newly delineated roles (e.g., agent or representative, advocate, ambassador, executor, intermediary, negotiator, proctor, promoter, steward, deputy, emissary, resource manager). Relational partnerships are built with equity, wherein the value of each participant is based on contributions to the relationship, rather than on positions within the healthcare system.

Although staff nurses are key to *recruiting* other nurses, nurse managers are key to *retaining* them. Collateral and equity-based process models of shared governance define employees by the work they support rather than by their location or position in the system. For example, the manager in the servant leader role retains nurses by providing human, financial, and material resources, support, encouragement, and boundaries for the staff nurse in the service-provider role. Staff nurses, then, are accountable for key roles and critical patient care outcomes around practice, quality, and competency.

Shared governance requires strategic change in organizational culture and leadership. It demands a significant realignment in how leaders, employees, and systems transition into new relationships and responsibilities. It begins with the definitions and objectives and flows from the shared governance process design.

# Chapter 2

# Design a structure to support shared governance

## Learning objectives

After reading this chapter, the participant should be able to do the following:

- Describe four elements that are essential to the successful implementation of shared governance in the earliest stages of process development.
- Discuss the basic guidelines for forming the governance bodies in shared governance.
- Compare and contrast four structural process models of shared governance.

*"Never tell people how to do things. Tell them what to do and they will surprise you with their ingenuity."* —George S. Patton

Every model, structure, or process of shared governance looks different when appropriately implemented at each level of the organization. The unique character of the organization, its mission, and its staff will create a process that reflects the nursing practice and leadership in that organization. However, some features of shared governance are similar enough to provide some guidance in designing a structure to support shared governance (Porter-O'Grady 2004; Peter 1991). (See the bibliography for many other excellent resources for designing and implementing a shared governance process model.)

All shared governance structures have certain characteristics in common:

- There is no one way to design or structure a shared governance process model.

- Shared governance is grounded in clinical practice.

- Nursing staff are responsible, are accountable, and have authority over all decisions related to nursing practice (practice, quality, and competence).

- Staff nurses are elected to the positions they hold in the shared governance structure by their peers rather than by management.

- Shared governance needs to be implemented *service-wide*, rather than unit-by-unit.

- Staff nurses define unit-based operational processes in the unit.

- Staff nurses drive the structuring of the shared governance process.

- Management, in the servant leader role, provides the support, encouragement, resources (financial, human, and material), training, and boundaries (organizational and management) necessary for success.

- A coordinating group composed of staff and management provides guidance about issues affecting the department of nursing, communicating the organization's strategic plan, developing shared governance bylaws, approving departmental expenditures or budgets, and/or helping determine accountabilities for appropriate groups/members within the shared governance structure.

- It is *responsibility* and *accountability based*, defined by what nurses do, how they do it, and the outcomes expected from nursing practice at point of care.

- Shared governance is *bylaws* or *rules driven*.

Effective shared governance does the following:

- *Transforms* the organization to a practice model of shared decision-making in a decentralized relational partnership with individual professional responsibility, accountability, and authority over practice decisions at point of service.

- *Empowers* the staff in unexpected ways, such as nontraditional involvement in operations and decision-making.

- *Shifts* some of the *accountability*, historically or traditionally part of the management role or owned by the organization, to staff nurses.

- *Shared decision-making* means many participants undertake multiple essential roles upon which each partner depends.

- When shared governance is implemented effectively, it affects the organization as a whole, *division-wide* **and** *unit based*.

## Basic requirements of all governance systems

Four elements are essential to the successful implementation of shared governance in the earliest stages of process development:

1. A *committed nurse executive* must be invested in process empowerment and must be willing to undertake the efforts necessary to implement shared governance.

2. A *strong management team* in terms of commitment to one another, to nursing, to the organization, and to the implementation process must exist.

3. The process cannot be implemented if employees do not have a *basic understanding of shared governance* and if they cannot build on that understanding with a working knowledge of what is to be accomplished. There must be a clear destination.

4. The *plan and timeline for implementation* are critical for charting progress points.

Governance systems are composed of governance bodies. Consider the following guidelines when implementing these bodies:

- A decision-making group is empowered to make decisions that form a baseline for thinking organizationally.

- The *group should be of an appropriate size (7–10 participants; generally no more than 14–15)* to facilitate effective group decision-making.

- Decisional groups must be *accountability* based.

- Within the organization, *all groups, committees, and task forces must relate to governance bodies or councils.*

## Structural process models of shared governance

In the past 35 years, four structural models of shared governance have emerged in the United States (Porter-O'Grady and Hinshaw 2005, Anthony 2004, Green and Jordon 2004; Hess 2004, Porter-O'Grady 1986, 1987, 1991): (a) congressional, (b) councilor, (c) administrative, and (d) unit-based. All four are based on essentially the same principles but reflect differing specific characteristics depending on the intention of the model, the design and structure of the organization, and the services building it.

### 1. Congressional model of shared governance

One of the first models developed, the *congressional model* of shared governance, primarily reflects a specific nursing orientation. This model features a staff congress composed of an elected president, a cabinet or senate of officers, and all the professional staff, including management and staff nurses, who oversee the operations of a unit, area, or department. The various *committees of congress*, who are delegated by the congress to make certain decisions and to have certain powers, are selected out of that congress and report back to the cabinet or senate. The congress defines its accountabilities and assigns them to various committees of the congress. See Figure 2.1 for a diagram of the congressional model (adapted from Porter-O'Grady 1991).

Five basic accountabilities emerge from the committees of congress: practice (P), quality assurance/improvement (QA), professional development/education (E), research (R), and

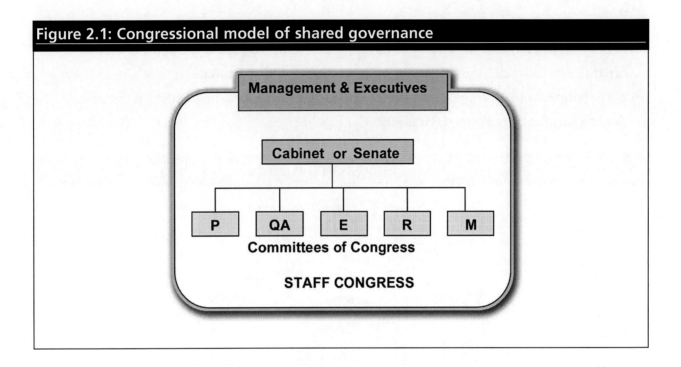

Figure 2.1: Congressional model of shared governance

management (M). These accountabilities reflect the disciplines' basic professional accountabilities. The nursing organization's work is carried out in the committees of congress.

## 2. Councilor model of shared governance

The *councilor model* is very similar to the congressional model. It consists of councils on
clinical practice, quality assurance, and staff development/education. Nursing staff empower these councils to perform the basic accountabilities identified in the congressional
model: practice, quality assurance/improvement, research, staff development/education,
and management. However, the structure is slightly different. Councils, as opposed to committees of congress, are empowered with the authority. Each council is delegated by the
organization with accountability and authority for decisions that fall within the context of
that council. For example, all practice decisions belong to the practice council, all quality
assurance/improvement decisions belong to the quality council, all professional development and education belong to the professional development council, and so on.

With the exception of the management council, all councils are made up predominantly of
staff nurses. They make the decisions related to accountabilities for practice, quality, and
competency that are staff-based. In that way, actual accountability shifts from the traditional management framework to a staff framework, as determined by the locus of control or

the legitimate place of that accountability. For example, practice should always be in the hands of the practitioners; therefore, practicing clinicians who are at the point of service or care make practice decisions. Responsibility, authority, and accountability for those decisions, policies, and outcomes rest with them. See Figure 2.2 for a diagram of the councilor model (adapted from Porter-O'Grady 1991).

## Figure 2.2: Councilor model of shared governance

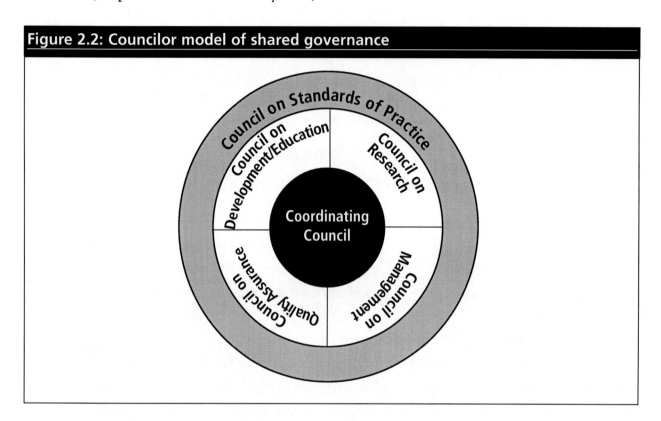

## 3. Administrative model of shared governance

The **administrative model** follows more traditional organizational lines of management and practice, with each having separate groups that address specific functions and accountabilities. The model resembles a more traditional hierarchy, with two structural units—management and clinical—that are generally aligned in a top-down relationship, although the members in both tracks may include both managers and staff as implementation advances. All work is done by committees and reported back to the overarching council or committee. The executive committee may make decisions on information provided for all clinical issues that concern more than one committee along either or both tracks. See Figure 2.3 for a diagram of the administrative model (adapted from Porter-O'Grady 1991; Hess; 2004).

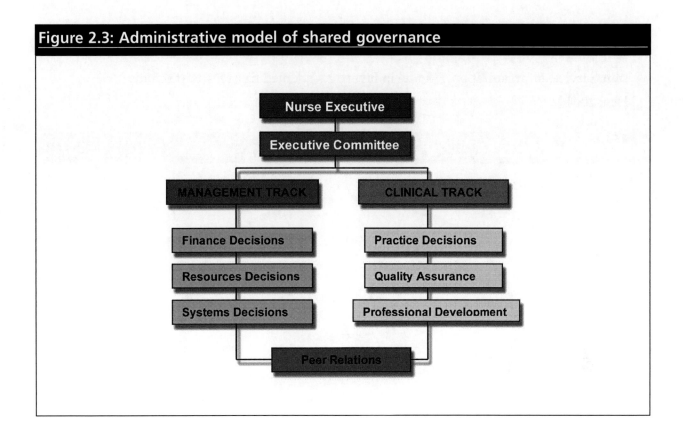

## Figure 2.3: Administrative model of shared governance

Communicating decisions upward is a key characteristic of this model. The decision-making groups are composed of at least 50% staff or of a representative proportion of staff to management, depending on the degree of organizational commitment to staff nurse participation in shared governance.

## 4. Unit-based model of shared governance

The *unit-based* model is rarely used. Note: This structural model is not to be confused with the *unit-based councils* in the councilor model. The design principles are similar but the structure is fundamentally different. The *culture* of the unit gives it form. Members define their own basic accountabilities. Units become entities unto themselves and make decisions about what they do and how they do it. These decisions may not affect the organization outside of the unit.

One of the problems with this model might be in its individual cultural application of shared governance, with no integrating or coordinating principles from the division as a whole giving it guidance. Individual units may build powerful decision-making models that staff nurses exemplify and appreciate, but it may jeopardize the structures of the whole division, service, or organization. (Model in Figure 2.4 adapted from Porter-O'Grady 1991; Hess 2004.)

## Figure 2.4: Unit-based model of shared governance

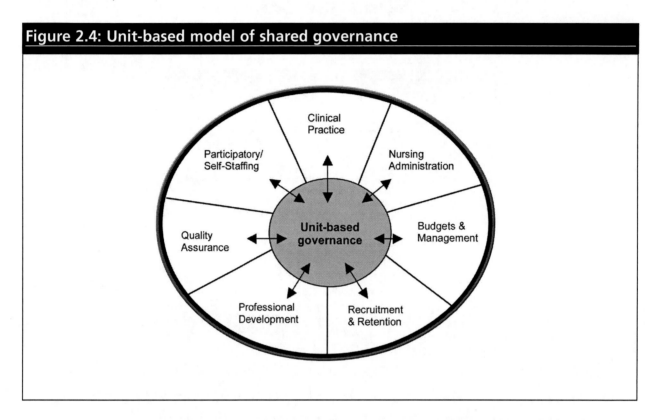

Shared governance demands an investment of effort and time by all partners in the healthcare system. As nurses reshape the professional practice community, the necessity for a relational partnership between management and staff nurses in decision-making affects the design and structuring of care in the professional practice environment. In the process, knowledge of the basic concepts and a commitment to them are prerequisites to implementation.

# Chapter 3

## Implementing shared governance

---

### Learning objectives

After reading this chapter, the participant should be able to do the following:

- Identify four strategic changes related to implementation of shared governance.

- Outline the three brain barriers to viable change in healthy organizations and the keys to overcome them.

- Describe the roles and responsibilities of a design team for implementation of shared governance.

- Discuss the purpose of bylaws and articles and how they are established when formalizing the shared governance structure.

---

*"The greatest amount of wasted time is the time not getting started."*
—Dawson Trotman

Venner Farley (2000) observed, "For nurses, re-structuring means change . . . Nurses must have a great capacity for change in order to accept the challenges of creating our future. The rewards will be substantial: autonomy and independence within a framework of collaboration and colleagueship." She encouraged nurses to begin thinking and behaving differently as they embrace change along five parameters:

1. Face reality as it is

2. Be open and honest with everyone

3. Lead, don't manage

4. Change before you have to

5. Recognize that nursing and nurses must seek and maintain a competitive advantage

**PART ONE**

## Leading strategic change

*"One of the reasons people don't achieve their dreams is that they desire to change their results without changing their thinking."* —John C. Maxwell

The changes in pace, demand, technological complexity, and patient populations today are greater than ever before. Consequently, the costs of resisting those changes and failing to implement collaborative partnerships in shared decision-making can be catastrophic. Specifically, nurses have choices about where and how they will work. They are no longer willing to work for authoritarian top-down management systems; instead, they are choosing ANCC Magnet Recognition Program® status hospitals with high-involvement shared governance processes and evolving professional nursing practice models. Strategic changes related to implementation of shared governance include structural changes, organizational changes, cultural changes, and individual changes (Porter-O'Grady, 2004), such as those listed in Figure 3.1.

## Figure 3.1: Four types of strategic changes related to implementing shared governance

### Structural changes

- Multidisciplinary work flow patterns
- Communication structures
- Ongoing assessment of work patterns
- Access to resources
- Investment at all levels of the organization
- Increasing dependence on interdependence
- Role definitions and descriptions
- Movement away from status determinations
- Based on accountabilities, not hierarchies

### Organizational changes

- Salaried work roles
- Reward systems; achievement rewards
- Gainsharing strategies
- Role accountabilities clarification
- Partnerships
- Mentoring and precepting roles
- Variable loci of leadership roles
- Work design (nurse driven)
- New orientation and socialization processes

### Individual changes

- New realities
- Degrees of change
- Sound practice standards
- Clear and strong ethics
- Dialogue and communication
- Honesty and integrity
- Curiosity and creativity
- Willingness to seek/abide by consensus
- Able to express concerns and ideas
- Structured risk taking
- Competency
- Varying degrees of involvement
- Increasing self confidence

### Cultural changes

- Reward systems altered
- Continuous management development
- Continuous leadership (manager and staff) development
- Career enhancement programs
- Hiring and termination processes
- Staff role ownership, including position descriptions
- Benefits programs
- Unit/service programs vs. divisional ones

A fundamental part of undertaking the processes associated with implementing shared governance and achieving successful outcomes is grounded in leading strategic change (Black and Gregersen 2003), which becomes the driving force for defining and restructuring professional relationships. Every decision and action is based on some idea or theory that events or actions will result in predetermined outcomes. These mental maps—or beliefs about cause and effect—guide people's decisions and behaviors. Most mental maps are forged in experience.

When people work successfully together in particular ways to make recurrent decisions and complete repetitive tasks, they begin to assume that the way they work is the ways things should be done. These decisions work well—except when things change. Black and Gregersen (2003) offer insights for changing mind maps that prevent people from changing or from maintaining changes, which is one of the greatest obstacles to implementing shared governance in professional practice settings. To tackle this problem, focus on changing the individual. The organization will follow.

Change is not easy. It begins and ends with employees' mental maps about the organization and their jobs. If those maps cannot be rewritten, if the brain barrier cannot be broken, there is nothing new for hearts and hands to follow. Staff-centered, patient-focused, relationship-based care in shared decision-making at point of service will not be possible.

This resistance to change is fundamental and biologically hard-wired into humans. We are programmed for survival, to resist random change, and to maintain stability and sameness. Black and Gregersen call this the "map-hugging dynamic." This dynamic occurs frequently among nurses who encounter shared governance for the first time; they may have difficulty letting go of old maps and ways of doing things.

Another element of this issue to consider is that fundamental change processes or cycles are based on the 80/20 principle, which says that 80% of the work comes from 20% of the workers. This explains why so many change initiatives fail: only 20% of the employees capture 80% of the picture of strategic change.

Black and Gregersen identify four stages of successful strategic change:

> Stage 1: Do the right thing and do it well.
>
> Stage 2: Discover that the right thing is now the wrong thing.
>
> Stage 3: Do the new right thing, but do it poorly at first.
>
> Stage 4: Eventually do the new right thing well.

Leading strategic change in reshaping professional nursing practice through shared governance and the essentials of magnetism (McClure and Hinshaw 2002) requires organizations both to channel efforts into training, educating, and empowering others to get ahead of the change curve and to master anticipatory change rather than subject themselves constantly to reactionary or crisis change.

## Overcoming 'brain barriers'

So how exactly does remapping change work? Black and Gregersen (2003) discuss three primary brain barriers that lead to failed change, as well as the keys to successfully overcoming those barriers and delivering strategic change in healthy organizations:

1. **Brain barrier: failure to see the need for change when what they have already been doing seems to still be working for them**

   - **Contrast.** Look at key contrasts. How are strategies, structures, cultural values, processes, technologies, practice models, and approaches to nursing leadership that worked in the past no longer effective in the present or appropriate for the future?

   - **Confrontation.** Leaders may have to confront nurses with clear and compelling evidences between past, present, and future contrasts to help them see the need before they can move to change. They cannot—and will not—change if they do not see the need to do so.

2. **Brain barrier: failure to move after they see the need to change because they do not believe in the new path, their ability to walk it, or the rewarding outcomes of the journey and destination**

   - **Destinations.** Make sure that all staff see the destination clearly to help them believe in the move to shared governance. People cannot change if they do not see the destination clearly or understand where they are going.

   - **Resources.** Give them the skills, resources (e.g., human, financial, material), and tools they need to reach the destination and participate in shared governance.

- **Rewards.** Deliver valuable rewards along the journey that have meaning to the employee. People value many things. The ARCTIC assessment tool (see Figure 3.2) can help identify rewards that would have greater meaning to people and more power to move change and successfully implement shared governance (adapted from Black and Gregersen 2003).

| Figure 3.2: ARCTIC assessment tool | |
|---|---|
| **ARCTIC** | **Potential rewards** |
| **Achievement** | • **Accomplishment:** the need to meet or exceed goals, to improve outcomes, and complete tasks successfully<br><br>• **Competition:** the need to compare performance, skills, abilities, and knowledge with that of others, to excel in comparison |
| **Relations** | • **Approval:** the need for favorable regard, to be appreciated and recognized by others<br><br>• **Belonging:** the need for connectedness, to feel like part of and accepted by an individual or group |
| **Conceptual/ Thinking** | • **Problem solving:** the need to challenge problems and find acceptable solutions<br><br>• **Coordination:** the need to link, adjust, relate, harmonize, integrate, and synthesize parts into a whole |
| **Improvement** | • **Growth:** the need to continuously develop and improve as a person and as a professional nurse<br><br>• **Exploration:** the need for discovery; to investigate systematically or to examine processes, evidence, and outcomes |
| **Control** | • **Competence:** the need for adequate or greater knowledge, skills, and ability to feel comfortable in doing a task or a job<br><br>• **Influence:** the need to contribute to, sway, or change others' opinions and actions; need or desire to produce an effect on practice and patient care outcomes |

### 3. Brain barrier: failure to finish because they are tired and lost

- **Champions.** Trained and motivated change champions are needed close to the action in every practice setting, from the moment that the decision to change is implemented.

- **Charting.** Progress must be measured at all levels in the organization and re-ported. Performance—good, bad, or indeterminate—needs to be communicated to staff members. Successful change requires monitoring and communicating at the individual level.

In summary, leading strategic change by breaking the three brain barriers involves remapping old behaviors and guiding staff through the process individually first in order to affect the organization as a whole. *Failure to see* is a problem of entrenched, successful maps that take high contrast and confrontation to break through this barrier. *Failure to move* happens when people resist going from doing the wrong thing well to doing the right thing poorly. It takes ensuring the destination is clear, resources are in place, and valued rewards are provided to break through this barrier. Finally, *failure to finish* is a consequence of nurses getting tired and lost and therefore not going fast enough or far enough. Champions and open communication about progress, good or bad, is critical for breaking through this barrier.

Change is constant. Indeed, it is the only real absolute in healthcare. Shared governance cannot be successful until all partners come together on how to lead strategic change.

**PART TWO**

## Shared governance systems: Perspective and format

Structure the shared governance format and vision carefully. Identify organizational and nursing's purposes, objectives, goals, direction, and strategic plan; reflect on the organization's mission; and determine the roles that nurses and nurse leaders will have in shared governance (e.g., conceptual base, philosophy, objectives, care standards, performance measures, quality assurance/performance improvement, professional development, and practice).

## Designing the shared governance process

Select members from nursing service and interdisciplinary teams to form a shared governance design team (or forum, group, steering committee, or coordinating group). They will obtain feedback from leadership and staff; consider nursing's objectives and the organization's goals, mission, and philosophy; and draft a process model for shared governance. Nursing staff and nursing leadership will select the final design to represent an integrated process and structure for shared decision-making toward positive patient outcomes. The structure and process should address each part of professional nursing practice: quality, competence, and practice.

Although there are four basic structures for shared governance described in the literature, the councilor model illustrated in Figure 3.3 is currently the most popular model used in nursing practice at point of service (Porter-O'Grady 2005, 1991; Anthony 2004; Hess 2004). Therefore, it will be presented in greater detail in order to develop the concepts and principles of shared governance implementation more fully.

## Implementing a councilor model for shared decision-making

To implement a shared decision-making model, you must do the following:

- Design a framework in which to discuss implementation of shared governance and set the direction for reshaping professional nursing practice.

- Evaluate the basic structure of the selected model (in this case, the councilor model).

- Identify and simplify accountability of disciplines. Five basic constructs can be separated or combined in the design structure of the governing councils or bodies. All professional committees, tasks forces, and practice groups will eventually be folded into one or more of these disciplines and become part of a designated governing council.

- Create a professional overlay for designing individual elements of the structure. The *accountabilities* (practice, management, quality, professional development/ education, and research) will be the basis of the formation of the governing councils, whether in five councils or in some other designated grouping.

**Figure 3.3: Councilor model governing councils**

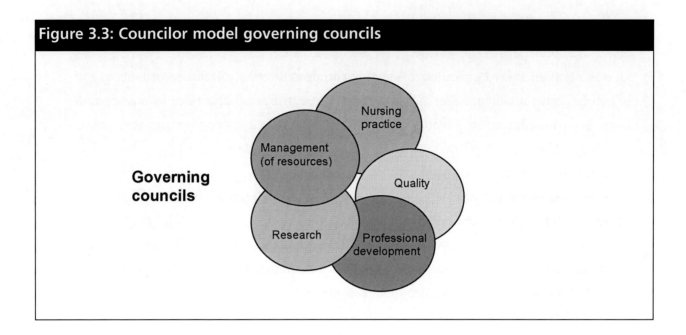

## Establish a design team, steering group, or coordinating group

a. **Design team size** (limit size to about 7–15 members)—The larger the group, the less constructive it may be in reaching consensus for making and implementing decisions.

b. **Design team membership**—The design-team mix needs to represent the percentage distribution of the organization of management and staff nurses (i.e., the majority). Drawing from services rather than from work units generally establishes a broader group but keeps the team small enough to be effective. Select nurse leaders, staff nurses, and interdisciplinary team members so they become partners in designing, implementing, and communicating the process elements of shared governance from the beginning.

c. **Design team purpose**—Focus on designing the shared governance process structure that will evolve after implementation:

- The entire design process falls under this group

- This team coordinates all of the shared governance activities initially

d. **Design team goals**—The team is empowered to do the work:

1) **Plan shared governance**—Define and describe what shared governance is and what it will look like in this organization at the point of service for nurses and nursing leaders. Identify the roles of the interdisciplinary team members, executive leadership, and internal and external stakeholders.

2) **Guide implementation**—Once the structure is designed and shared governance has been defined in terms of an implementation plan, the design team continues to guide the process. Over time, the design team may change names (e.g., coordinating council, nursing assembly, or nursing forum) and expand functions to facilitate the ongoing progress of shared governance in nursing.

3) **Help nursing staff and leaders with transition**—Create a timetable for transition. Assess readiness. Complete predetermined activities and provide subsequent activities for group members once councils are established. Develop a mechanism for personal and professional transitioning, a way of acknowledging accomplishments, and a social or symbolic activity for the transition (Porter-O'Grady 2004).

4) **Evaluate progress**—Evaluate progress initially, at six months, and then annually once shared governance is implemented. Include where you are, how far you've come, and what has to be done in light of the design or plan you set in motion. Doing so is critical to measuring success (Hess 1998).

## Roles and responsibilities of the design team

a. **Learn about shared governance and how it works**—If they are responsible for designing the format for shared governance, they need as much knowledge as possible from the beginning stages through mature development and standardization of practice. Build an information base to understand and structure the work.

b. **Select a shared governance process structure or model**—Determine which shared governance structure or model applies to the organization based on its culture, goals, and strategic plan. The structure must be a good fit for the organization and for professional nursing practice. Expect this structure to be adapted initially and multiple times as it matures and conforms to the needs of the nurses and the organization, with more and more voices represented over time.

c. **Identify tasks and create a timeline**—Focus on what will occur at progress points along a time line to evaluate elements of the process and to ensure that everyone succeeds in finishing assigned tasks. Developing this process is a long-term event. It usually takes three to five years to fully implement an effective, efficiently operating shared governance process model. Each stage of the process builds on previous stages. Therefore, evaluate each stage before beginning the next stage. Let the timeline become a guide to implementing the process successfully and to determining where you are along the way. It helps keep the destination visible so that all participants can move to accept and manage the many changes needed for shared governance (Black and Gregersen 2003; Porter-O'Grady 1991).

d. **Evaluate goals and process outcomes**—Emphasize goals and anticipated outcomes at the beginning of the process (e.g., higher levels of nurse satisfaction, higher retention rates, increased patient safety outcomes). Measure and evaluate goals intermittently along the way. Design or select tools for measuring progress in shared governance that allow for evaluation and adjustment in the process as outcomes are achieved.

## Designing governance councils

When establishing the selected shared governance process structure, identify how many councils (bodies or groups) will be created to include all five accountabilities or disciplines. Once the disciplines are accounted for, there is no right or wrong way to design the structure or process. One organization chose to create five governing councils: (a) nursing assembly (management/coordinating council), (b) practice council, (c) quality and research council, (d) professional development council, and (e) unit-based councils, which were connected to each of the other four councils. This approach allowed nursing to slightly reduce the number of council meetings staff nurses would need to attend while still maintaining representation in each governing body. (In this book, a council is described separately for each accountability or discipline for the purpose of discussion.)

Begin by identifying the outcomes desired. Establish one council at a time. Doing so will help employees transition more easily and successfully through the change process.

a. **Start with the management (coordinating or leadership) council**—Purpose and responsibilities: Provide guidance and linkage to the governing councils, and serve as a mechanism for the nurse executive, nurse leaders, and nurse managers to participate in activities related to the provision of nursing care at point of service. The management council deals almost exclusively with resource issues and allocations. The role for nurse leaders and managers in shared governance is primarily servant-based, providing resources, support, opportunities, boundaries, and protection (i.e., from losing needed resources for staff nurses during annual budget allocations) for nursing staff at point of care, thereby freeing staff to focus all of their experience, expertise, and effort on caring for the patient and improving patient care outcomes. The manager does the following:

- Appropriates necessary resources for the professionals in practice (human, fiscal, material, support, and systems)

- Centers service around the practicing professional at point of care

- Integrates (links) the shared governance process with the other services and roles

- Channels information to and from staff nurses through unit-based councils to and from nursing and organizational leadership, when appropriate

- Identifies systems problems and generates necessary responses

- Communicates encouragement, support, and boundaries (e.g., tells staff nurses when there is no budget for new equipment requested by the unit-based council, and then helps them explore other options for getting the necessary resources)

Management frequently has the most growth and change to undergo for shared governance to be successful. Empowered staff members assume new roles of responsibility, authority, equity, accountability, and ownership traditionally belonging to managers, which can cause territorial, personality, and role conflicts. Nurse leaders will need educational programs to help them adapt to new behaviors, learn new roles, and develop new skills as their current role evolves from management to servant leadership, a much higher, more powerful, and more demanding form of leading. This process will be challenging for them. Devoting time and resources to their transitional development in the transformation of their leadership roles is critical.

b. **Establish the unit-based councils**—This usually follows or correlates well with the implementation of the management council. Here is where it all comes together. Purpose and responsibilities: to promote autonomy, equity, partnership, and shared accountability and ownership for unit operations by managing point-of-service care; measuring and documenting patient outcomes (nursing quality indicators); providing orientation, mentorships and/or preceptorships for new employees, new graduates, and students doing clinical rotations; participating in schedule development; sharing charge nurse responsibilities; conflict resolution and problem solving; assessing and meeting educational needs and unit-specific competencies; engaging in evidence-based practice (research, journal clubs); monitoring unit-specific practice and safety issues (policies, quality improvement, patient safety); and managing unit education (inservices, mandatory training, continuing education).

c. **Develop a practice council**—Purpose and responsibilities: to set the criteria for evidenced-based practice consistent with established/evolving professional standards and regulating agencies. This council keeps the development of the staff in concert with the changes of management/leadership roles. Most of the other councils' work will depend on the foundational work completed and managed by the practice council, which has the control and authority to make decisions affecting policies and practice for the work that they do. A practice council does the following:

- Defines, implements, and maintains practice
- Selects theory base
- Sets practice standards
- Sets performance standards
- Defines career advancement

d. **Initiate a quality council**—Purpose and responsibilities: to monitor and evaluate performance and outcome measurements based on evidence-based practice using the best scientific knowledge available, to provide a forum for interdisciplinary team collaboration, and to integrate quality initiatives into practice. The work of the quality council depends on the work of the management and practice councils. For example, the practice council's service standards need to be developed before the quality council can identify and develop measurement standards. Performance standards must be done before developing a performance evaluation system (quality council). Therefore, establish a deliberate, step-by-step relationship among the councils and a framework to support their complementary development.

The goal of shared governance is that ownership and investment of all the workers and the outcome of the work ties back into how we define the work and how performance is measured against that definition. If staff members define the work, perform on that definition, and achieve work outcomes, they also can evaluate progress or individual performance related to that work. A staff member does the following:

- Monitors and measures standards of care.
- Designs the quality and performance improvement system.
- Controls the performance evaluation system (a peer-based process in shared governance, not management-based).
- Sets the goals for patient care monitoring (defines a standard of care, measures it, reaches it, and changes the standard so nurses work at a higher level of function or outcome).
- Manages the credentialing and privileging program. Every professional nurse has an obligation for the quality and type of work each one does. Establishing a peer-based process for new nurses when they first enter the organization that continues throughout the nurse's employment helps ensure a good fit with the organization and with nursing service.

e. **Initiate nursing professional development council**—Purpose and responsibilities: to provide orientation; to assess ongoing learning and competency needs; to define, implement, and maintain standards, continuing education, and inservices that promote professional and personal growth and ongoing competency of professional nurses and their healthcare team members.

- Ensures professional competency in ongoing learning activities, the basis of performance measurement over the long term. This council facilitates implementation of competency mechanisms that ensure a continuous mechanism for education and development is present, is staff-based, and clearly represents the work done, rather than representing some pre-planned objective that may or may not reflect the unit-specific needs of the nurses at point of service.

- Develops an effective communication network through each of the councils.
- Manages staff orientation programs and preceptorships, which are critical to the success of new employees (graduate nurses, nurse managers, agency/contract nurses), and manages unit-specific or clinical orientations.
- Facilitates staff nurse development though credentialing, certifications, and academic advancement.
- Plans quarterly and annual staff meetings:

  (1) **Quarterly meetings:** Staff and council members deal with issues of concern to the organization as a whole as it affects nursing service; report to staff what activities they've been involved in and get feedback from the staff about what is occurring; relate, communicate, and interact; look at goals and learning objectives for the year, review activities and the progress of those activities over time, and deal with operational issues.

  (2) **Annual meetings:** Staff and council members look at goals and objectives of the organization, discuss/report the annual learning needs assessment and education plan, consider problems and issues of the discipline (education and professional development) as a whole, determine how to fit those issues with the goals of the organization, and review organizational problems and issues affecting the discipline. This is an opportunity to give awards for service and to acknowledge the contributions of those who have acted on behalf of staff during the previous year. It can be an opportunity for formal and informal communication and celebration.

- Facilitates nursing staff members' access to learning-teaching activities by bringing training to the unit level. Balance, personal growth, and professional development are natural outcomes of shared governance activities. Facilitating unit-based education is a major goal of this council. The learning process, content, and activities become more real and meaningful when applied directly to professional practice at the point of service.

f. **Establish a research council (if applicable)**—This council follows the development of the previous two councils addressed, the quality and professional development councils. Not all organizations have well-defined research activities, but research is one of the clinical accountabilities in shared governance and is part of the Magnet Recognition Program journey. Professional nurses need to be committed to validating old knowledge and discovering new knowledge, which is an integral part of the research process. Research seeks knowledge that will enhance patient care outcomes and offer a new basis for the work to be done at point of service. It helps staff nurses develop critical thinking skills, evidence-based practices, and abilities to understand and participate in research at the point of care. This council is a way to formalize that process. It is the last council implemented because it depends on the other councils being in place and is the most resource-dependent council.

## Focus on council membership

When recruiting members for the shared governance councils, consider factors such as representation, contributions, membership mix, size of councils, length of time of participant service, and meeting times.

a. **Representation**—especially from a service context. These representatives will speak on behalf of those services when decisions have to be made.

b. **Contributions**—by each member that grows over time; work may be assigned to members to be done in the meeting or to be taken back to their units/areas and completed there. Reports on tasks and progress are given at each council meeting.

c. **Membership mix**—Staff governance councils (practice, quality, professional development) need to be composed mostly of staff nurses, about 70%–90% clinical staff. The other council members should be management or support staff. These are staff nurse councils. They will make staff decisions that affect clinical practice, quality, and competency. Messages of empowerment, equity, autonomy, and accountability are delivered in an effective and clear way so that shared decision-making emerges in the partnership between staff and management.

d. **Size of councils**—Number of participants depends on the number of units represented.

Usually, only 7–15 members are recommended. However, some organizations have more representatives at the table. All nursing units/areas should have someone at the table to represent their voices in the discussions and shared decision-making. Keep in mind, however, that the larger the group the more difficult it is to get consensus and make decisions. You would have to address this issue at the beginning of work in larger groups.

e. **Length of time of participant service**—It often takes about a year for a participant to learn the roles of assigned councils. Therefore, a two-year term seems to be emerging as the standard length of service commitment for each council member. With such a term, consider rotating half of the members off one year and the other half off the second year. This rotation would provide continuity of process, with at least one-half of the members every year having served for one year and being able to orient and mentor the incoming council members.

f. **Meeting times and structures**—How organizations elect to structure their council meetings and times will depend on factors unique to that staff.

- Some councils meet once a month for eight hours (a full day) to accomplish the tasks of the council. This approach allows members to focus on the business of the council instead of dividing their attention with concerns about the patients or tasks they left on the unit for an hour or two.

- Other councils have a monthly "Meeting Day" when all councils meet, usually for an hour each, at different times to allow staff members to attend their meetings and return to work around the council meetings. Breaks of 15–30 minutes between council meetings allow staff members who serve on more than one council to get to the next one without disrupting or interfering with the work of other councils. A schedule of such a day might look like this:

    **8am–9am** Management or Coordinating Council
    **9:30am–10:30am** Quality Council
    **11am–12pm** Professional Development Council
    **12:30pm–1:30pm** Practice Council
    **2pm–3pm** Research Council

- Council meetings **cannot** be optional. Attendance has to be mandatory if staff nurses and nursing leadership are to have a voice in shared decision-making and if they are to be able to complete and communicate council activities. It is **critical** that nursing leadership support and facilitate staff attendance at assigned council meetings. It is also important to provide time and opportunity for communication of information and/or data gathering to complete council assignments (e.g., unit inservices). Each nurse leader/manager and his/her staff should discuss and resolve these details from the beginning.

Each council is structured with certain accountabilities or disciplines. Staff councils must identify the authorities that belong to the staff and operate within the staff framework.

## Focus on a shared governance empowerment process

Each governing council selects a chair from among the membership to provide leadership for the council. For the staff councils, that chair will be selected from among the staff. The research council chair may be management or staff, and the management council selects its own chair. These chairs must be empowered to manage or lead the councils with the responsibility, authority, equity, ownership, and accountability to make decisions and to act on those decisions. Empowering the chair means the chair of each council will be given certain basic powers secured by the role. It is recommended that the chair do the following:

1. Be elected by peers.

2. Control the agenda.

3. Act for the group, speak for the group members, and make decisions for them when the group is not in session.

4. Assign group tasks/functions.

5. Move the group to decision-making when discussion indicates a need.

6. Accept no additional assignments. This role is extensive enough on its own.

7. Remove non-performing members from the group if necessary.

# Chapter 4

## The roles of the stakeholders

---

### Learning objectives

After reading this chapter, the participant should be able to do the following:

- Discuss the roles of the following four stakeholders in shared governance: leadership, union representatives, community members, and patients.

---

*"No significant learning occurs without a significant relationship."*
—James Comer, MD

For shared governance to succeed, a consortium of stakeholders must participate in it: researchers, administrators, nurse executives, staff nurses, interdisciplinary team members, patients, and community members. Their roles are as diverse and interrelated as their expertise, experiences, and education. Four such stakeholders, or partners, include leadership, union representatives, community members, and patients.

## Leadership partners in shared governance

Shared governance helps those in leadership positions—administrators, nurse executives, nurse managers, and supervisors—step back from many tasks and decisions about practice, quality, and competency that staff nurses are more than qualified to make. Nurse leaders provide a professional practice environment that supports and facilitates staff nurse autonomy, equity, ownership, and accountability.

## Union partners in shared governance

Although a complex system with many guidelines and regulations, the simplified purpose of the union in most healthcare organizations is twofold:

1. To provide collective bargaining to help nurses gain control over their practice and accomplish professional and economic goals, objectives, and outcomes

2. To protect nurses from demanding or unfair management standards that threaten the quality of nursing care or negatively affect the professional practice environment (e.g., unsafe or ineffective staffing ratios, mandatory overtime, and unsafe or hostile work environments, among others)

Even though both collective bargaining and shared governance are about giving nurses a voice in decision-making in ways that affect practice at the point of service and organization-wide, shared governance is **not** collective bargaining. Shared governance **is** shared decision-making.

The goal in shared governance is to integrate collaborative practice into the professional practice environment through shared decision-making. By partnering with the union representatives in the healthcare organization from the beginning, the interdisciplinary team members can communicate this intent and address concerns and issues as they arise, thereby increasing understanding and reducing or eliminating the confrontation that sometimes occurs in such discussions (Porter-O'Grady 2005).

## Community partners in shared governance

Nurses engaged in shared governance often partner with members of their communities in activities that reflect positively on the organization and nursing service. They share in the decision-making about which activities to support and to provide. Community collaborations include those with staff nurses participating in outreach programs, such as the following:

- Offering a CPR Day for the community members each year

- Presenting a health fair annually with staff nurses, who negotiate the vendors and activities for various patient populations from the community (e.g., prostate cancer screenings)

- Obtaining affiliations with local universities and colleges for nurses to continue their academic educations on hospital grounds

- Allocating and using appropriate resources to support various projects (e.g., a Junior Internship Program that brings high school students into the organization during the summer and teaches them how to communicate and interact with patients)

## Patients as partners in shared governance

Patients today are very knowledgeable and unwilling to be directed in their treatment plans. They want a voice in what treatment approaches will be implemented, which medications they will take, and where they will be hospitalized. Shared governance is an integrating structure (Porter-O'Grady 1991) that pulls together all the participants: nurses, physicians, interdisciplinary team members, patients, and family members. As a process structure of partnership between staff nurses and patients, shared governance provides a vehicle for improved communication, greater responsibility and accountability, and a way of coordinating, integrating, and facilitating care at the point of service.

Patients respond positively when staff nurses partner with them in their care decisions. Some staff nurses make walking rounds during shift changes and intermittently throughout their shifts. They stop to speak with their patients each time and ask for their feedback, questions, concerns, and ideas. If the doctor came by earlier, the nurses ask the patient what was said and listen to his or her report instead of telling the patient what the physician wrote in the chart or told the nurse. These staff nurses invite patients to attend the interdisciplinary team meetings when the team members are discussing that patient's care. Engaging patients in conversation is one method of involving them in their own care. When staff nurses interact relationally with patients in partnership, patient and nurse satisfaction scores increase.

# Chapter 5

## Nursing's role in organization-wide shared governance

---

**Learning objectives**

After reading this chapter, the participant should be able to do the following:

- Discuss nursing's role in organization-wide shared governance related to the process structure or model, other disciplines and departments, and corporate and organizational integration.

- Describe how shared governance can be an integrating structure in healthcare organizations under nursing leadership.

---

## A multifaceted role

Nursing's role in organization-wide shared governance is multifaceted:

- **Shared governance is a universal process structure or model.** It can be applied in any setting. As it emerges in one division, it begins to affect other services, departments, and disciplines that want to participate in decisions that affect their future and roles or to be involved to the fullest extent possible. That is to be expected and anticipated.

- **Implement in other departments and disciplines when they are ready.** Although nurses generally lead the process change, shared governance will vary in terms of organizational application. When other departments are ready, nursing must be ready to assist, to encourage, and to act as role models by sharing the information and experiences gathered in their own implementation process. Allow the shared governance process model to evolve in the divisions, disciplines, and departments that seek it.

- **Structure corporate and organizational integration into the shared governance process.** Nursing support gives the organization an opportunity to integrate everyone's growth in shared governance. Healthcare systems can only change strategically if the whole organization joins nursing's efforts and they collectively institute the necessary structures for change together. Shared governance needs to be incorporated so that it becomes an organizational imperative and continues to grow across the organization.

## How shared governance can be an integrating structure in healthcare organizations

Many organizations have developed institutional process models (Porter-O'Grady 1991), where all disciplines and departments have some role in making decisions that affect the direction and the operation of the organization. As individual disciplines do their work, they integrate with this larger process model. All employees play a role in the organization as a whole by participating in the directions, policies, decisions, and objectives that set the organization on a course for its own future. Nursing has an opportunity to lead organizations into that future through shared governance.

Shared governance process models and institutional models take on numerous designs to provide a framework for members, divisions, and departments of the whole organization to participate in seeking goals and objectives that guide their future. Organizations with such models must emerge and begin to lead the direction of the whole organization by providing a framework for integrative process models and shared decision-making.

Shared governance should be an integrating structure (Porter-O'Grady 1991, 2005), then, one that pulls all the participants together. It is a structure of partnership between manager and staff; between organization and discipline, division, and profession; and between employee and organization. It provides a vehicle for change, ownership, equity, investment, partnership, accountability; and a way of coordinating, integrating, and facilitating the work of healthcare today and tomorrow.

One fundamental aspect of shared governance is the need to join all parties in a venture to which they are fully committed. The structural process and the emergent system will provide an integrative structure for collectively moving the organization toward desired outcomes and strategic change.

The next step in implementing a shared governance process is to continue gathering information and resources to design, implement, and evaluate your own shared governance process. This book is designed to provide a broad base upon which to build planning and implementation. Although there is no "right" process model, the basic principles of shared governance are generic and viable.

# Chapter 6

## Assess your process

---

**Learning objectives**

After reading this chapter, the participant should be able to do the following:

- Discuss the research project that looked at shared governance in a
  government agency using the Index of Professional Nursing
  Governance (IPNG).
- Describe the six dimensions measured by the IPNG.

---

*"Additional problems are the offspring of poor solutions."*
—Mark Twain

Assessments and measurements of shared governance process models range from case study exemplars and implementation stories to research-based studies. Anthony (2004) provides an excellent overview of many of these studies. Anthony's anecdotal evidence with subjective evaluations of outcomes provides a road map for designing and monitoring governance structures.

## Measurement tools: IPNG and IPG

To evaluate the distribution of governance (see Appendices A and B), Hess (1998) developed and validated an 86-item measurement instrument. He contends that because outcomes are never measured with changes in governance, no evidence exists to connect them. However, his tool has been used in more than 50 hospitals, is presently being used in at least six research endeavors and 10 reported research studies. More than 20 ANCC Magnet Recognition Program® status hospitals have used Hess' tool to evaluate their progress in developing and/or establishing shared governance. It is currently the most-used instrument for measuring governance to date. The vast majority of research-based studies evaluate shared governance in single settings, using either cross-sectional or longitudinal time frames.

Hess's Index of Professional Nursing Governance (IPNG) has been used to measure governance in healthcare organizations for more than 10 years. IPNG evaluates the implementation of innovative management models and tracks changes in governance (see Appendix A). The more global index, Index of Professional Governance (IPG), measures the perceptions of all healthcare professionals within an organization (see Appendix B). These instruments are reprinted in appendices with permission.[1]

Implementing a shared governance nursing practice model changes the organizational culture. Nursing shared governance moves any organization from a hierarchical structure in any form to a unit-based, councilor, administrative, or congressional structural form that requires ongoing interdisciplinary collaboration, communication, flexibility, evaluation, and redesign of goals and processes.

---

[1]The subscales keys, which are necessary to interpret the IPNG and the IPG, are available for a nominal charge to researchers, clinicians, and administrators who formally request permission and agree to adhere to guidelines for use. Free use of the instrument may be available for graduate students and researchers, particularly those conducting outcomes investigations. Revenue generated from the use of the IPNG and IPG is used to support the work of the Forum for Shared Governance and the development and maintenance of its Web site, *www.sharedgovernance.org.*

## Research on the principles of shared governance

*"Destiny is not a matter of chance, it is a matter of choice; it is not a thing to be waited for, it is a thing to be achieved."* —William Jennings Bryan

For those interested in learning more about the research and work done over the past 30 years on shared governance and leadership, some excellent articles and books are available from the fields of business, management, economics, human resources, and healthcare. Anthony, Hess, Kennerly, Porter-O'Grady, and others have studied the principles of shared governance and found them to be accurate delineators of nurse empowerment (Porter-O'Grady 2003, 2005). They and their colleagues have investigated multiple theoretical and empirical evidences to define shared governance and to determine whether a shared governance nursing practice model based on the principles of partnership, equity, accountability, and ownership achieves the positive outcomes desired.

## Research on shared governance in a government agency

Hess and his colleagues (Howell et al. 2001) used the IPNG to study an established shared governance process model within a government agency, a highly bureaucratic and hierarchical management system. They defined nursing governance as

> multidimensional, encompassing the structure and process through which professional nurses in healthcare agencies control their professional practice and influence the organizational context in which it occurs . . . [and] loosely described shared governance as a system of structuring nursing practice that gives nurses at the bedside the responsibility for decisions related to their practice. In the words of Prater, it "implies the allocation of control, power, or authority (governance) among mutually (shared) interested and vested parties." (pp. 187–188)

### Six dimensions for measurement

The researchers studied 183 registered nurses in Nursing Service at the Durham (NC) VA Medical Center (273 surveys were distributed but only 183 returned). They used the 86-item instrument IPNG to measure nurses' perceptions of professional nursing governance facility-wide on a continuum ranging from *traditional* (dominant group is nursing management/administration) to *shared* (decision-making shared between staff nurses and management/administration) to look at six dimensions with subscales:

1. **Nursing personnel**—who controls nursing personnel by hiring, promoting, evaluating, recommending, adjusting salaries and benefits, formulating unit budgets, creating new positions, conducting disciplinary action, and making terminations.

2. **Information**—who has access to information relevant to governance activities: opinions of managers, staff nurses, physicians, patients, and interdisciplinary team members; unit budgets and expenditures; nursing service goals and objectives; and the organization's finances, compliance reports, and strategic plan.

3. **Goals**—who sets goals and negotiates resolution of conflict at different organizational levels among nurses, other members of the interdisciplinary healthcare team, and organizational leadership: philosophy, goals, objectives, and formal grievance procedure.

4. **Resources**—who influences the resources that support professional practice: monitoring and securing supplies, recommending and consulting other services, determining daily assignments, and regulating patient movements (admissions, transfers, referrals, placements, and discharges).

5. **Participation**—who creates and participates in committee structures related to governance activities: committees that address policies and procedures for clinical practice, staffing, scheduling, budgeting, and collaboration.

6. **Practice**—who controls professional practice: patient care standards, standards of professional practice and care, quality, staffing levels, qualifications, competency, professional development and education requirements, and evidence-based practice (incorporating research into practice).

Higher scores on any of the six subscales indicated that nurses perceived themselves to have greater influence over professional decision-making in their organization. Three of the six dimensions (nursing personnel, information, and goals) were consistent with traditional governance strategies, although the scores on information and goals were very close to the shared governance range. In the other three dimensions, nurses perceived a significant shift toward shared governance in areas of resources, participation, and practice at near or higher than the base range. The results of this study demonstrated that "shared governance within several critical areas of nursing practice can be successfully implemented" (Howell et al. 2001).

Further research using valid instruments, such as the IPNG, must examine outcomes associated with varying levels of implementation of shared governance and its role in the recruitment and retention of nurses. As medical care is integrated into healthcare systems, community-based outpatient centers, and cybertechnologies that triage and treat patients across cyberspace, staff nurses are becoming more involved in shared decision-making. What impact will shared governance have on the professional practice environment of care for new generations of nurses in a sociotechnological era?

# Chapter 7

# Case studies: A snapshot of shared governance on large and small scales

## Learning objectives

After reading this chapter, the participant should be able to do the following:

- Compare the attributes of a shared governance process in organizations of different sizes and settings.

### Introduction: The shared governance process in organizations of different sizes and settings

Shared governance takes on different shapes in various organizations because of the unique culture of each institution. However, if organizations remain true to the principles in their design, implementation, and evolution, then they share the basic elements, or attributes, of shared governance—they are just rolled out in different ways. For example, this chapter details the inner workings of shared governance in two vastly different hospitals. Consider how the process is similar despite the difference in size and setting.

## Case study #1: Saint Joseph's Hospital, Atlanta

### Background

Saint Joseph's Hospital (SJH) in Atlanta is a 410-bed tertiary care hospital. In the late 1970s and early 1980s, due to the repercussions of relocation and increased competition, SJH's nursing vacancy rate hovered at nearly 20% and turnover around 35%. Patient satisfaction was low, and quality was problematic in some areas. We needed a fresh start.

SJH's journey toward developing a distinguished nursing organization began when the nursing division implemented shared governance as the professional practice model (PPM). The decision to implement shared governance resulted from a commitment to make SJH a place where nurses could work with significant autonomy.

### Implementation

Knowing that nurses desired control over practices and procedures that affected direct care, we identified several priority areas in our search for a structure, including education, quality assurance, management, and standards for practice. These four areas served as the basis for our original shared governance councils.

### *Education council*

*Responsible for professional development*

- Arranged educational programming for the units
- Developed educational programs for practice changes
- Created patient education materials

### *Quality assurance council*

*Responsible for comparing nursing practice to current standards and determining the rate of compliance*

- Coordinated ongoing compliance measurement activities
- Made suggestions to standards about deficits in practice

## Management council

*Nursing leadership is responsible for securing material fiscal and human resources and for enforcing compliance with work developed by the three staff councils*

- Secured adequate staffing and determined staffing matrices based on patient needs
- Budgeted for nursing care

## Nursing standards council

*Responsible for nursing process assessment, plan, intervention, and evaluation*

- Developed standards, policies, and procedures that govern nursing care
- Developed the care delivery model

## Best practices to handle the nitty-gritty

### Determining council membership

The council model was developed by a team of staff and nursing leadership. Once the council structure was determined, membership criteria needed to be developed and members selected. Prospective members for the staff councils completed applications for membership (just as we do today) and were selected by the development team. Today, the council members select the new members. Currently, members are selected for a two-year term and rotate in either October or April, thus limiting the amount of turnover at one time. The chair and vice chair each serve for two years, so the longest possible term one can serve on a council is six years. Once the nursing division council model was assigned and implemented, each nursing unit was expected to develop a similar structure.

When they were formed, the councils had eight to 12 members. As the model matured, these members were often forwarded for membership by their respective unit-based governance committees. On the staff councils, only the staff RNs could vote with a leader serving as an advisor. CNSs were also assigned to a council for support, without voting privileges. Also, the councils asked other hospital professionals to serve in

C
A
S
E

S
T
U
D
Y

#

1

advisory, non-voting capacities (e.g., the hospital quality assurance/performance improvement coordinator serves as an advisor to the nursing quality assurance council). Councils also invited other hospital staff to attend council meetings, as needed (e.g., nursing informatics staff are invited to standards council meetings to determine online charting practices).

### Ensuring staff involvement in council activities

Council members represented several areas to control the size of councils and to enhance the council's ability to develop an effective team. Initially, motivation among peers and replacement of RNs who spent time off the unit to participate in council activities fueled involvement in shared governance. At the time, the usual workday was eight hours, so a staff council member was paid eight hours to participate in council day. The council meetings usually lasted about six hours, with the other two hours for council work completed outside the council meeting.

Due to the significant commitment required of the council chair, the council chair was paid for two eight-hour days each month and was also freed from clinical responsibilities during these times. The chair's manager must ensure that he or she is relieved of bedside responsibilities during the council meeting.

In 1985, the standards council developed and implemented a clinical ladder/levels advancement process. In developing the ladder, this council awarded points for various activities that support shared governance. Council membership grew so popular that the bylaws had to specify that a period of six months had to elapse before applying for membership on another staff council.

### Developing leadership skills

Ensuring competency among council leadership was then and remains today the greatest challenge to the shared governance model. To address leadership competency and at the request of staff nurses, the "vice chair" position was developed to help inculcate understanding of the necessary leadership abilities of council chairs. Various programs were developed to help with leadership development (e.g., leadership classes, team leading). Each council also has a leadership advisor who does not vote but who is present for leadership mentoring.

**C
A
S
E

S
T
U
D
Y

#

1**

## Closing the communication loop

A year after all of the councils started, it became clear that there was a lack of communication between councils, especially as there were no shared members (e.g., no staff member could be a member of more than one council at a time). This difficulty in "closing the loop" led to the creation of the coordinating council. This council is made up of the chairs of each shared governance council and a handful of other nurse leaders. A staff nurse elected by peers chairs this committee. The coordinating council was responsible for coordinating council activities, setting the nursing strategic plan, developing and revising the nursing staff bylaws for annual staff vote, and preparing the staff to select the guiding nursing theory for nursing services.

## An evolving process[1]

Until 2004, there were relatively few changes made to the initial council structure, which included changing council names (see Figure 7.1), modifying supporting councils, and increasing council responsibilities.

---

### Figure 7.1: SJH's governance structure

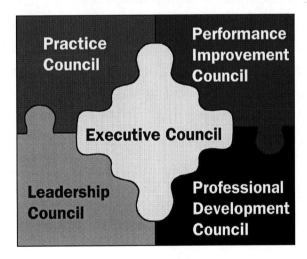

*Source: Saint Joseph's Hospital, Atlanta. Reprinted with permission.*

---

[1]Partially adapted from Sharkey, K. (2005). "Embody nursing excellence through change: Why a designated hospital aligned its ppm with the 14 Forces." *HCPro's Advisor to the ANCC Magnet Recognition Program*, 1(8), 7–8. HCPro, Inc.

**C A S E   S T U D Y   # 1**

When SJH first developed its shared governance model, it created a nursing research forum as a subcommittee of the nursing performance improvement council. Nurses of all educational levels who supported nursing research within the facility served on this subcommittee. Although this structure was effective at the time, SJH recognized the need to assess our PPM's infrastructure continuously to keep it energized and focused in the face of emerging challenges.

Therefore, in 2004, the nursing division aligned its own strategic plan with the organization's strategic plan to focus on completing both nursing and hospitalwide goals. Several of the strategic initiatives developed for nursing focused on research projects and, because SJH is an ANCC Magnet Recognition Program® (MRP) designated organization, increasing staff awareness of how the Forces of Magnetism applied in their daily practice. For the first time in 25 years, SJH made a significant change within its PPM by eliminating the nursing research forum and expanding the PPM to include a sixth independent council devoted to nursing research.

Last year, the executive council, which sits at the core of the PPM, made the motion to change the bylaws to create that sixth council. The staff nurses voted to accept this change. SJH redesigned the conceptual model of shared governance to portray the relationship that the research council would have with all the other councils. To complete the process, each council was aligned with the Forces that it best represents. This new model is the focal point of discussion during nursing orientation because it clearly depicts the interrelation between our PPM and the tenets of the MRP (see Figure 7.2).

## Figure 7.2: Revised governance structure

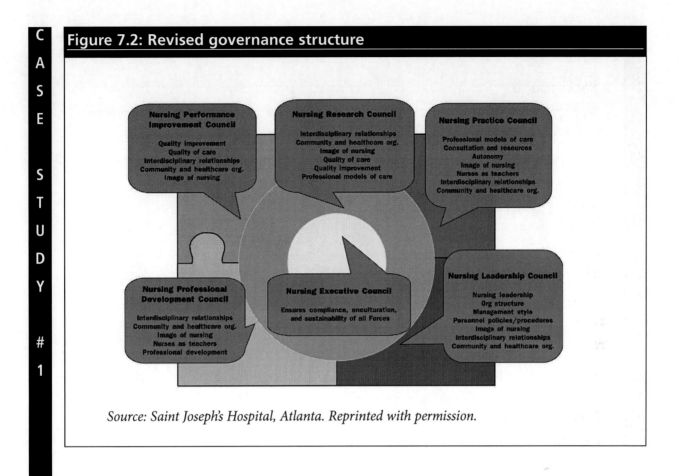

*Source: Saint Joseph's Hospital, Atlanta. Reprinted with permission.*

In 2005, we celebrated our 25th anniversary of shared governance. Members of the nursing staff have remained vigilant over the years to ensure that our model holds true to the concept of shared decision-making. Decisions about direct care must remain in the hands of those who provide it, although it is not always easy to discern where responsibility for all types of decisions lies.

Looking back over the years, we are struck by the elegance of the SJH shared governance process model, which was implemented by Sharon Finnigan and Tim Porter-O'Grady when they were newly appointed nurse leaders at SJH. Their energy and enthusiasm not only generated interest and restored a sense of pride to much of our nursing staff at the time of implementation, but it also inspires us to ensure that shared governance flourishes in our nursing environment over time, and throughout change.

C A S E   S T U D Y   # 1

## Case study #2: Southwestern Vermont Medical Center (SVMC), Bennington

### Background

As part of its journey to elevate the professional role and recognition of the registered nurse, SVMC—a 99-bed community hospital in rural Vermont—undertook an ambitious campaign to decentralize the nursing department and empower the direct care RN. One step in that process was the development and implementation of a shared governance model of professional practice.

In 1994, SVMC formed a shared governance steering committee, consisting of RNs from each nursing unit, two nursing directors, and the CNE. The steering committee explored models of shared decision-making and became interested in Tim Porter-O'Grady's councilor model of shared governance. Convinced that this model would support the goals established by the steering committee, Porter-O'Grady was invited to present his model to the nursing staff at SVMC. More than 60 nurses attended the program, and it gave the staff the vision and energy they needed to move forward with the development of their shared governance model.

### Implementation

The shared governance model that was implemented in 1994 mirrored the Porter-O'Grady model, as described in his book, *Implementing Shared Governance: Creating a Professional Organization* (1992). It consisted of four primary councils—practice, management, education, and quality—and a coordinating council, which facilitated the communication between the other four councils.

Membership within the practice, education, and quality councils included staff nurses from each of the nursing units and a nursing director. A staff nurse chaired each council. The management council included all of the nursing directors, the CNO, four staff nurses, and a nursing director who served as the chair. The coordinating council's membership included the chairs of each council in addition to the CNO, who served as chair.

## Original structure and responsibilities

The original roles and responsibilities of each of the councils are described in the following sections.

### *Practice council*

A. Role: The professional practice council defines the parameters of clinical practice. It is the primary decision-making body related to clinical issues within a professional framework.

B. Responsibilities: The function of the professional practice council includes but is not limited to the following:

1. Standards of care and practice: To oversee the development, implementation, review, revision, and approval of standards of care and practice at SVMC, including, but not limited to, procedures, protocols, and guidelines.

2. Clinical advancement: To oversee the clinical advancement program and provide direction for structure, finance, and the appeals process.

3. Peer review: To review the process of evaluating professional accountability, including, but not limited to, peer review, job descriptions, and performance appraisals.

4. Delivery of care: To provide direction for delivery of care.

5. Resource utilization: To make recommendations for resource utilization (e.g., staffing, budget, product selection, capital purchases, and professional development).

6. Information systems: To collaborate with nursing information systems on issues that interface with nursing practice.

## *Management council*

A. Role: The management council supports, facilitates, and integrates the mission, vision, and values of Southwestern Vermont Health Care (SVHC), our corporate organization, with the philosophy of professional nursing practice.

B. Responsibilities: The function of the management council includes but is not limited to the following:

1. Development, implementation, review, and revision of nursing department policies.

2. Establishment and maintenance of practices that ensure fiscal viability in a managed care environment.

3. Development and implementation of cost accounting systems to achieve cost reductions.

4. Identification of staff learning needs to facilitate practice in a managed care environment.

5. Establishment and maintenance of staffing patterns to meet the needs of defined patient populations.

6. Integration of the JCAHO and other regulatory agency standards into practice.

7. Oversight of the development and implementation of patient care standards.

8. Appointment of nursing representative(s) to the employee participation committee.

9. Participation in the development of the SVMC strategic plan.

10. Establishment of annual nursing department goals to achieve the SVHC strategic plan, the hospital's annual operational objectives, and the continued development of professional practice.

11. Support of the SVHC/SVMC mission, vision, and values through program and service development.

### Education council

A. Role: The education council provides direction for nursing education to promote optimal professional competencies.

B. Responsibilities: The function of the education council includes but is not limited to the following:

1. To identify long- and short-term educational goals.

2. To facilitate education related to quality issues and practice issues.

3. To facilitate communication related to new products, pharmaceuticals, and new policies.

4. To facilitate communication of unit-based educational programming and competencies.

5. To maintain communication with the multidisciplinary education committee.

6. To meet with nursing educators who use the hospital as a clinical site at least annually to influence curricula and to improve learning experiences.

C
A
S
E

S
T
U
D
Y

#
2

*Quality council*

A. Role: The quality council oversees and coordinates nursing PI/CQI activities to support the SVMC mission, vision, and values and annual performance improvement plan using an interdisciplinary approach.

B. Responsibilities: The function of the quality council includes but is not limited to the following:

1. To establish monitors for identified patient care and nursing practice standards to ensure compliance.

2. To evaluate monitors that continue out of compliance for more than one quarter.

3. To act as a resource and provide education for unit-based quality improvement functions.

4. To perform root-cause analysis for all nursing sentinel events.

## Refining the vision

In 1997, three years after the shared governance model was implemented at SVMC, the first major modifications to the program occurred. At the coordinating council's annual review of the professional practice bylaws, which define the shared governance model, staff discussed their feelings of a disconnect between the management and practice councils. Nursing procedures were developed, reviewed, and revised at practice council, but the supporting policy was the responsibility of management council.

Staff also expressed a desire to have a stronger voice in areas that governed the professional work environment, such as scheduling, staffing patterns, and vacation time. At this meeting, a decision was made to merge management and practice councils into one and to name this new group the leadership council. The membership for this council included a staff nurse representative from each nursing unit, all nursing directors, and clinical nurse specialists.

C
A
S
E

S
T
U
D
Y

#

2

## An interdisciplinary shift

In 1999, the second major change in the shared governance model began. The need for greater interdisciplinary collaboration in clinical practice was becoming apparent. To support the goal of having all clinical departments work together to drive best patient outcomes, it was decided to move to an interdisciplinary model of shared decision-making. The chief nursing officer was also the chief operating officer, with responsibility for all clinical departments, which facilitated this move. The revision of the shared governance model into an interdisciplinary model was recognized as a significant change, requiring buy-in from the other clinical areas as well as from nursing. The transition of the councils was set to occur over a one-year period, with one council at a time moving to the interdisciplinary structure.

## New structure and responsibilities

The process was completed in early 2002, taking a little more time than anticipated. The new council structure and responsibilities are described in the following sections.

### Leadership council

A. Role: The leadership council supports, facilitates, and integrates the mission, vision, and values of SVHC with the philosophy of professional nursing practice. It defines the parameters for clinical practice and is the primary decision-making body related to management and clinical practice.

B. Responsibilities: The function of the leadership council includes but is not limited to the following:

1. To develop, implement, review, and revise nursing department policies, procedures, standards of care, guidelines, and protocols to meet JCAHO and other regulatory guidelines.

2. To establish and maintain systems that ensure fiscal viability.

3. To provide input and leadership in the development of the strategic plan.

C
A
S
E

S
T
U
D
Y

#
2

4.  To provide direction for clinical advancement and peer review process.

5.  To provide leadership and direction for evaluation and modification of the care delivery system.

6.  To provide direction and guidance for the selection and implementation of nursing information systems.

7.  To work collaboratively with the department of human resources on recruitment and retention activities.

8.  To appoint nursing representative(s) to employee participation committee.

9.  To establish annual nursing department goals to achieve the SVHC strategic plan, the SVMC's annual operational objectives, and the continued development of professional practice.

10. To ensure that nursing procedures are developed, reviewed, and revised in an evidenced-based process, using current research, standards of care, and best practice findings. Existing procedures are reviewed and revised as necessary every three years, or more often as needed, per JCAHO standards.

    a.  The procedure review committee is operationally accountable to the leadership council. The procedure review committee, through leadership council, has access to the resources needed to ensure that the most current evidence and literature are available for review.

    b.  Membership of the procedure review committee includes representation from each nursing unit. The committee is chaired by a clinical nurse specialist and meets at least quarterly.

    c.  Specialty-specific procedures are developed, reviewed, and revised at the unit level. Appropriate resources to support the evidenced-based approach are available through the unit-based budgets.

## Clinical education council

A. Role: The clinical educational council serves as the mechanism for defining educational needs throughout the hospital. As needs are defined, the educational council will ensure that individuals/departments create programs/plans to meet the identified needs.

> The council is responsible to the director of education for ensuring compliance with regulatory requirements and other education-related mandates.

B. Responsibilities

   1. To establish educational priorities based on regulatory requirements and identified learning needs.

   2. To ensure compliance with mandatory educational programming.

   3. To oversee implementation of departmental education plans.

## Clinical quality

A. Purpose/Function: The clinical quality council oversees and coordinates nursing and other clinical performance improvement activities to support the hospital's mission, vision, and values and to uphold the functions of the hospital's performance improvement plan using an interdisciplinary approach. As such, the council does the following:

   1. Establishes, reviews, and/or helps to revise monitors for identified patient care and nursing practice standards to ensure compliance.

   2. Evaluates monitors that are out of compliance or below threshold for more than one quarter to ensure that there is an adequate corrective action plan to make and sustain improvement.

**C
A
S
E

S
T
U
D
Y

#
2**

3. Acts as a resource to provide education for unit-based and departmental quality-improvement functions.

4. Evaluates trends and coordinates efforts to make recommended improvements.

5. Reports on trends, findings, improvement opportunities, and accomplishments through representation on the hospital's PI committee.

### Coordinating council

A. Role: The coordinating council ensures the overall coordination of the activities of the other councils and is accountable for the integration of services and decisions that affect the nursing department and other clinical departments. The coordinating council will integrate the SVHC mission, vision, and strategic goals into the nursing department plan.

B. Responsibilities: The function of the coordinating council includes but is not limited to the following:

1. To review monthly minutes from all councils.

2. To ensure two-way communication to all councils, staff, and administration.

3. To problem-solve issues referred by councils.

4. To review professional practice bylaws and nursing department plan of care annually.

5. To support the development and implementation of unit-based councils.

6. To monitor ongoing progress toward achievement of department goals.

C
A
S
E

S
T
U
D
Y

#
2

## Shared governance in action

The interdisciplinary focus of the professional practice model of shared decision-making has improved communication and collaboration among all disciplines. Physician leadership recognizes the leadership council as the decision-making body for the clinical departments and uses this council to develop patient care protocols, medical staff policies, and physician orders. For example, when the pharmacy and therapeutics committee (which is a medical staff committee) decided to develop a glycemic control protocol, it used leadership council for input into nursing and pharmacy's responsibility within the protocol. This collaboration allowed for the creation of a protocol that respects the roles and responsibilities of each clinical department.

As another example, the chair of clinical quality reported on the lack of progress by individual nursing units to reduce medication errors at coordinating council. Recognizing that it needed to address medication errors from a broader perspective, the coordinating council established a medication error task force, which included staff nurses, a nursing director, and the director of pharmacy. This group conducted an in-depth analysis of medication errors and reported back to leadership council with recommendations on system changes to improve the safe administration of medications.

## An evolving process

The shared governance model of professional practice at SVMC has continued to evolve and mature. Each nursing department has developed its unique unit-based model that supports the larger model. All nursing units and most of the other clinical departments have self-scheduling models in place. Staff nurses are responsible for the shift-to-shift adjustments in staffing based on their professional knowledge and judgment as to the care needs of patients. An example of how one unit has continued to evolve its shared governance model is the Peer Support Team (PST) developed by SVMC's women's and children's unit. The purpose of the PST is to resolve issues or conflicts that arise between staff regarding professional behavior/conduct before the matters require intervention from the department director. The PST consists of three staff nurses—one from each shift—who are selected by their peers. Educated on conflict management and negotiation, the team approaches each case referred to them with the intention of

**C**
**A**
**S**
**E**

**S**
**T**
**U**
**D**
**Y**

**#**
**2**

resolving the issue so staff feel supported and respected. Nursing directors support the SVMC shared governance model, as it allows them to focus on broader organizational strategic initiatives. Nurses and other clinicians express satisfaction with their ability to voice concerns, put forth new ideas, and participate in decisions that affect both their clinical practice and the professional work environment.

# Chapter 8

## The relationship between shared governance and the ANCC Magnet Recognition Program®

---

**Learning objectives**

After reading this chapter, the participant should be able to do the following:

- Identify the two central elements of the ANCC Magnet Recognition Program® and the shared governance process.

- List the "eight essentials of magnetism" and how they compare to the shared governance process model.

---

*"I find the important thing in life is not where we are, but in what direction we are moving."* —Oliver Wendell Holmes

The mission of the American Nurses Credentialing Center (ANCC) is to promote excellence in nursing and healthcare globally through credentialing programs and related services, among which is the Magnet Recognition Program® (MRP). Some describe this program as the "Nobel Prize" of nursing excellence in professional practice environments.

The relationship between shared governance and the MRP is synergistic. *Shared governance* is a process form of structure for autonomous staff nurses to share their experiences and secure decision-making power in an organization. Shared governance asks, "What decision have you made lately?" Achieving MRP status is a cultural, transformational journey. MRP designation and shared governance must be a part of the strategic plan for the organization when nursing excellence is the standard of professional practice.

## Magnet Recognition Program® goals

The ANCC Magnet Recognition Program has three primary goals:

1. Promote quality of healthcare services in an environment that supports professional nursing practice

2. Identify excellence in the delivery of nursing services to patients/residents

3. Provide a mechanism for the dissemination of "best practices" in nursing services

The journey to designation shares two central elements with the shared governance process model: cultural enhancements and structural enhancements.

- *Cultural enhancements.* The work environment is changed during this process, enabling and empowering nurses at point of care to improve and enhance patient outcomes. The journey will not be successful without a culture of shared decision-making among professional nurses and the interdisciplinary team members (clinical and administrative) being in place first.

- *Structural enhancements.* A strategic plan is built around the autonomy of nurses to share decision-making and to function in four primary professional roles: clinical practice, education, research, and administration. Shared governance provides a professional practice environment in which nurses can develop and mature in these roles to enhance the organizational culture effectively.

## Benefits of designation and shared governance

Two groups of people are already reflecting and building the 14 Forces of Magnetism into their culture:

- Those who have implemented shared decision-making, professional nurse autonomy, and the essentials of "magnetism"

- Those who are putting the essentials in place and beginning to change the culture before demonstrating it through the application for designation

The benefits of MRP designation are reflected in effective shared governance, described by such nurse researchers as Havens and Aiken (1999) in Figure 8.1.

### Figure 8.1 Benefits of designation reflected in shared governance

**For the patient/client**

- Reduced patient mortality
- Reduced patient morbidity
- Increased patient satisfaction
- Increased patient safety
- Decreased "failure to rescue"

**For organizations**

- Decreased length of stay
- Decreased cost of nursing staff replacement
- Increased opportunity to market institution
- Variable costs of implementation

**For nurses**

- Lower nurse turnover
- Lower nurse vacancy rates
- Lower nurse "burn-out" rates
- Lower nurse emotional exhaustion
- Decreased needlestick injuries
- Better nurse-physician relationships
- Higher nurse satisfaction
- Decreased work-related injuries
- Higher nurse-to-patient ratio
- Decreased medical errors

Shared governance helps those in leadership positions provide a professional practice environment that supports and facilitates staff nurse autonomy in the following areas:

- Determining education credentials

- Evaluating and writing research

- Writing/updating policies and procedures

- Participating in scheduling

- Managing their own competencies

- Providing inservices and continuing education

- Precepting students/new graduates/new employees

- Any other duties they are interested in learning and participating in with their nurse management/leadership, interdisciplinary team members, and administration

## Essentials of "magnetism"

"Eight essentials of magnetism" are evident in every culture of shared governance and show what keeps nurses working in professional practice environments (McClure and Hinshaw 2002):

1. *Working with clinically competent nurses*—Staff nurses participate both in identifying their own competencies each year based on what's new, changed, problematic, and high risk in the practice environment and in verifying how they meet those competencies. They also collaborate with nurse leaders to identify and verify the organizational competencies that also need to be addressed.

2. *Good nurse-physician relationships*—Mutual respect exists between nurses and physicians.

3. *Support for education*—Advanced credentialing through facilitation and flexibility of work schedules and resources provided (e.g., bringing academic education onto the campus out of respect for the nurses' work-life balance needs).

4. *Adequate nursing staffing*—Participation in staffing schedules: engagement, involvement, and decision-making on the part of staff who are thinking beyond the unit to the organization as a whole.

5. *Concern for the patient is paramount*—Doing what is needed for the staff first (e.g., providing resources and ongoing training to maintain/enhance competency) so they can focus all their energy, expertise, and experience on meeting the needs of the patients, which is the essence of *staff-centered, patient-focused, relationship-based care.*

6. *Nurse autonomy and accountability*—Improving communication and delegation by bringing together partnership, equity, responsibility, authority, ownership, and accountability in shared decision-making in the professional practice environment.

7. *Supportive nurse manager/supervisor*—The nurse manager or supervisor is the key retention person at the point of care. This role is critical to effective outcomes related to shared decision-making and implementation of a shared governance process model at the unit and organizational levels.

8. *Control over nursing practice and environment*—In which shared decision-making leads to better patient outcomes and partnerships between patients and healthcare providers.

Shared governance pulls everything together and reshapes nursing practice to provide an environment of professional excellence that flows well through the Forces of Magnetism. Through ongoing nursing research and evidences of best practices, nurses excel in decision-making at the point of service. They enjoy collegial management and staff partnerships, collaborative practice among all members of the interdisciplinary teams, and accountability-based ownership in issues related to practice, quality, and competence.

## 14 Forces of Magnetism

If the Magnet Recognition Program is the Nobel Prize of nursing, the 14 Forces of Magnetism comprise its core and shared decision-making constitutes their expression in healthcare. The Forces are categories of attributes or outcomes that exemplify nursing excellence and are evidenced by shared decision-making, partnership, equity, responsibility, accountability, authority, and ownership in professional practice.

The 14 Forces of Magnetism (see Figure 8.2) are fundamental to determining excellence in the professional nursing practice environment. The MRP is about the journey. The Forces are based on compelling original research (McClure and Hinshaw 2002) and make it easier to engage nursing leaders and staff nurses in the process of shared governance and the journey to excellence—even if the organization is not going for designation.

---

**Figure 8.2: The 14 Forces of Magnetism**

1. Quality of Nursing Leadership
2. Organizational Structure
3. Management Style
4. Personnel Policies and Programs
5. Professional Models of Care
6. Quality of Care
7. Quality Improvement

8. Consultation and Resources
9. Autonomy
10. Community and the Hospital
11. Nurses as Teachers
12. Image of Nursing
13. Interdisciplinary Relationships
14. Professional Development

---

## Forces of Magnetism relative to shared governance

1. **Quality of nursing leadership**—The chief nurse officer (CNO) is a knowledgeable and strong risk-taker. He or she provides a professional practice environment and philosophy of mutual advocacy and shared decision-making within nursing service. The CNO sits at the highest decision-making place in the organization—at the senior management committee table—so that all nurses' voices can be heard throughout the organization and so their interests can be represented. The CNO, the ambassador for nursing service, protects nursing leaders and staff nurses from political and economic influences that could negatively affect patient care outcomes or the professional practice environment.

2. **Organizational structure**—Decentralized, flat organizational structure that creates a sense of partnership, equity, accountability, and ownership within the professional practice environment. Typically, the CNO reports directly to the chief executive officer (CEO) and serves at the executive level of the organization. Although the MRP has no criteria for how the organizational structure should look, a structure or process that is dynamic and responsive to change must be in place. A formal structure is critical to manage nurses' involvement through a representative model. Every organization

develops its models and cultures differently, but all of them include strategic planning, shared decision-making, and staff responsiveness. The organization demonstrates strong nursing representation in committee structures and through a functioning and productive system of shared decision-making.

### Best practice in a government organization

*"Leadership is practiced not so much in words as in actions."* —Harold Geneen

Joy Easterly, the Associate Director for Nursing Services/Patient Services at the Bay Pines (FL) VA Healthcare System, is a highly respected CNO who sits on the executive committee and represents nursing service at her organization's highest level. She shares in the decisions regarding the organization's strategic plan and nursing's role in its implementation. Easterly meets monthly with her nurse leaders (i.e., nurse executives, nurse managers, and clinical nurse specialists in nursing education) and briefs them on the goals, needs, and direction of the organization, especially as they affect nursing service. The nurse leaders are entrusted to do the following:

- Communicate the outcomes, suggestions, and information received at the leadership meeting to their staff nurses

- Solicit staff nurses' input, questions, ideas, and concerns

- Respond to any decisions staff nurses make or request related to the information relayed from the leadership meeting

- Represent staff nurses at the next leadership meeting

As with all government agencies, the VA struggles with a degree of hierarchical organizational structure that can limit shared decision-making throughout the organization (Howell et al., 2001). Nevertheless, Easterly has worked closely with nurse leaders and staff nurses to design an effective infrastructure that positions the organization for excellence in nursing service across the continuum of care and at the point of service.

3. **Management style**—The CNO and nurse leaders help staff nurses create vision, philosophy, and shared purpose through supportive discussion. Feedback is valued and communicated at all levels of the organization as appropriate. Staff nurse leaders are visible, accessible, and committed to working closely with the interdisciplinary team and other staff members. Nurse managers provide support, encouragement, resources, boundaries, and protection through shared governance in matters of practice, quality, and competence.

*Best practice in management style*

**Charge nurse program in shared governance**
Contributed by Ann Cellamare, RN, BSN, of the Bay Pines (FL) VA
Healthcare System

The entire RN staff on the surgical care inpatient unit was given the opportunity to rotate to the charge nurse position for one week. During that week, they were closely monitored by all disciplines, and evaluations (including a self evaluation by each RN) were given to the nurse manager. At the end of the rotations, three nurses requested to continue working in the charge nurse role. They met and identified the following areas as new responsibilities and accountabilities with appropriately designated authority to be developed and supported:

- Complete individual development plan (IDP) to give each new charge nurse a foundation upon which to build personal and professional goals.

- Develop interpersonal skills with all disciplines and interdisciplinary team members.

- Enhance each staff nurse's leadership ability and recognition among peers and higher management.

- Provide opportunity for advancement.

- Restructure the patient education delivery system.

- Work with the staffing coordinator on developing a team scheduling model and encouraging other staff nurses to participate in developing/contributing to their own schedules.

- All work will be evenly divided among the nurses. Each will assume his or her charge responsibilities for three to four months at a time and then rotate.

4. **Personnel policies and programs**—Staff nurses are involved in the decision-making about budgets, schedules, salaries, competencies, resources, and practice. For example, staff should be familiar with budgets and their roles and responsibilities related to organizational and unit stewardship. Salaries and benefits are competitive with community standards.

Creative and flexible staffing models and schedules accommodate the many demands that staff nurses experience on their time and attention at work and at home. Increased patient acuities and workloads require shared decision-making at the point of service to maximize staff satisfaction. For example, one innovative group of staff nurses worked with their nurse manager to restructure their shift hours. They showed how 12-hour shifts rotating from 7 am to 7 pm and 7 pm to 7 am was not effective for them. After some negotiation, staff nurses demonstrated how patient care outcomes supported their proposal positively and successfully changed their 12-hour shift rotations to 3 am to 3 pm and 3 pm to 3 am. The new schedule resulted in more enthusiastic and committed staff, fewer call-ins, and a deeper respect for nursing leadership and the process of shared decision-making.

5. **Professional models of care**—Nurses are accountable for their own professional practice and the model of care selected for their nursing service. Shared governance provides a process structure for assessments, strategic change, and ongoing evaluation of patient outcomes and care delivery models that promote professionalism, accountability, evidence-based practice, adaptation to regulatory needs, and a staffing system that reflects patient needs. Models of nursing care (e.g., relationship-based care (RBC) model) give staff nurses the responsibility, authority, and accountability (R+A+A) to provide and coordinate patient care at the point of service.

This Force can be confusing because it looks at which nursing theorists are used in the organization (e.g., Benner, Peplau, Neuman, King, or Orem). Can nurses talk about them (i.e., who are they, what are theorists needed for, and what is their purpose)? Professional care models provide a theoretical foundation on which to build research, contrasts, and comparisons. They form the basis of the discipline of nursing. Because there is no one theory that covers all patient populations with their unique needs, organizations usually adopt several theorists who blend into the conceptual framework and reflect values and philosophies of each unique nursing service.

Shared governance practice councils delineate the models of care and find evidence that they are hardwired into the organization and that nurses have adequate resources to accomplish desired patient care outcomes. Nurses need to know that they are all practicing under this standard. They also need to know the difference between care delivery systems and models of care. For example, team nursing is a *care delivery system*, or *nursing model of practice*. Rocchiccioli and Tilbury (1998) describe eight care delivery systems: functional nursing, team nursing, primary nursing, primary-team nursing, total patient care, modular nursing, differentiated practice, and case management. These are not conceptual models of care.

6. **Quality of care (Force 6)** and **quality improvement (Force 7)** are about structure and outcomes. Quality of care is about the effectiveness of the system to support nursing and patient care. Staff nurses engaged in shared governance make meaningful decisions about quality practice at the point of service. They are responsible for providing evidence-based care that is grounded in research and facilitates improved patient care outcomes.

7. **Quality improvement** (QI) is the process that advances the quality of care and services within the organization. It focuses on operational effectiveness and clinical processes and outcomes.

*Best practices in quality improvement through shared governance*

**Nursing case study investigations (CSI) in shared governance**
Contributed by Michelle Jans, MSN, APRN, BC, CNS, in Bay Pines (FL) VA
Healthcare System

The nursing CSI is a process for analyzing the events around patient outcomes that resulted in either near misses or medical errors of varying degrees. Each month, staff nurses develop case studies around real incidents that are identified through root cause analyses (RCA), incident reports, or tagged by nursing leadership/staff nurses as potential learning opportunities. Using a detective-like method of inquiry, staff nurses identify "clues" to the underlying problem(s) that may have changed the patient's outcome if they had been recognized earlier. They use this information to solve the case by doing the following:

- Diagnose learning needs

- Implement advanced assessment skills, critical thinking, and evidence-based inquiry

- Discover limited/incomplete data within policies that would help them provide a more appropriate clinical pathway to the presenting clinical picture

- Increase interdisciplinary team member communication and collaboration

- Improve documentation in content and context

- Enhance professional practice skills (organization, prioritization, delegation, problem solving)

- Engage in open and honest peer review

Through shared problem solving, the nursing CSI has become a forum where nurses can achieve a greater level of excellence by carefully considering the evidences in practice, evaluating the clues along the way, and finding successful solutions to the case at hand.

8. **Consultation and resources**—This Force is about cataloging local/national speakers brought in for training, nursing grand rounds, clinical nurse specialists (in consultative roles), experts and expertise available within the organization or made available by bringing in consultants, and field trips to other facilities to review/learn about best practices in nursing. The organization and nursing service provide adequate resources, support, and opportunities for these activities, many of which are identified by staff nurses throuogh their governing councils.

9. **Autonomy** is one of the fundamental principles of shared governance. Staff nurses within the organization govern their own practice and share in making decisions that affect practice, quality, and competence. They partner with other healthcare providers and patients to deliver care at point of service. Nurse leaders facilitate nurses' success by providing the resources, support, encouragement, and boundaries they need to dispense patient-focused care.

10. **Community and the hospital.** Healthcare providers build relationships within and among all types of healthcare and community organizations. They develop strong partnerships that support positive patient outcomes and the health of the local communities they serve. Nurses engaged in shared governance recognize and embrace their responsibilities to support community outreach activities that help both nursing service and the organization be seen as strong, positive, and productive community citizens. This is accomplished through community collaboration, positive outcomes from collaborations, and allocation and use of appropriate resources as needed.

*Best practice in community outreach*
Paul F. Sink, Jr., Nursing Education Coordinator, Nursing Home at James A. Haley VA Healthcare System in Florida, coordinates the continuing nursing education provided for a workshop on hurricane preparedness for Tampa and the surrounding communities each year. Sink is part of a multidisciplinary team of healthcare providers, safety specialists, and subject matter experts working to help citizens remain safe during the many hurricanes and tropical storms they endure each year.

11. **Nurses as teachers.** Nurses educate, precept, coach, orient, and mentor other nurses, students, and patients within the organization. They get involved in the lifelong learning of others, both inside and outside of their communities. Students from a variety of clinical and academic programs are welcomed, supported, and engaged in the organization. Affiliation agreements and contractual arrangements are mutually beneficial.

In a shared governance practice setting, leadership supports nurses and expects them to serve as educators/teachers to ensure the foundation for quality of care, a staff nurse domain, and ongoing competencies. Nurse development and mentoring programs prepare staff preceptors to work with all levels of students.

Nurses in all positions serve as faculty and preceptors for students and new employees. Staff nurses provide patient and family education, clinical and leadership development, inservices, and scholarly initiatives.

*Best practice for nurses as teachers through shared governance*

**Coordinators of unit education (CUE) in shared governance**
Contributed by Beatriz Rodriguez-Santiago, MSN, CNS, Nursing Education, Bay Pines (FL) VA Healthcare System

In this organization, a CUE is defined as *a staff nurse who is responsible for assessing, planning, coordinating, and evaluating the educational needs of the nursing staff at the unit level.* The CUE works closely with the clinical nurse specialist assigned to his or her unit, the charge nurse, and/or the nurse manager to track educational programs that develop and maintain staff competencies. They help staff nurses provide quality care to the unique patient population on their assigned units by creating a continuous learning environment. CUEs do the following:

- Identify the inservice education needs of the staff on the unit with the assistance and support of the CNS, nurse manager, and nursing staff

- Coordinate inservice programs

- Schedule speakers for varied inservices based on assessed needs

- Network with CUEs from other units/areas to share information and provide cross-training inservices when appropriate

- Publicize centralized nursing education learning activities

- Maintain accurate records of individual staff members' attendance in inservice programs, mandatory reviews, and external learning events

- Enter training data into the hospital education tracking system

- Help the nursing staff retrieve training data whenever necessary

Each month, CUEs attend meetings to discuss their roles and responsibilities and how their work fits into the overarching strategic plan for continuing nursing education and staff development within the whole organization. They hold a great deal of respect, autonomy, and mutual accountability with the nursing staff, which helps ensure the highest level of excellence in nursing care.

12. **Image of nursing.** Ask staff nurses to describe what MRP designation and shared governance mean to them. Build and expand the image of nursing within the organization and community. Recognize and reward nursing service's contributions. Ensure that other members of the healthcare team characterize nursing services as essential to the organization and integral to the overall well-being of patients. Make sure that staff nurses' voices are heard and respected in the governing councils, in other departments and divisions, and in their nurse-physician and interdisciplinary team member relationships, effectively influencing systemwide processes.

13. **Interdisciplinary relationships.** Shared governance creates a forum for staff nurses and interdisciplinary team members to develop and enhance mutual respect, knowledge, competence, and a platform for essential and meaningful contributions toward quality clinical outcomes. Collaborative working relationships within and among the disciplines are actively cultivated and valued.

14. **Professional development.** Successful nursing partnership, equity, accountability and ownership in practice demand lifelong learning. Examples of lifelong learning activities are listed in Figure 8.3.

---

**Figure 8.3: Examples of lifelong learning activities**

- Quality orientations

- Career development services

- Academic or formal education

- Continuing education

- Inservices

- Competency-based clinical and leadership/management development

- Career development

- Professional certification

- Continuous learning environment

- Sufficient human and fiscal resources for professional development

- Support of excellence in clinical practice and leadership

- Promote advanced practice and certification

- Build professional relationships and mentors

---

This transition to shared governance can be very difficult for nurse leaders and staff nurses. It is always easier to do the work yourself after so many years of having done it a particular way, especially if that approach has been successful. It is also very difficult to give over "management" duties and step back to monitor staff in doing the tasks with which they, the nurse leaders, are so comfortable. However, giving that authority and power to staff is critical to a mature shared governance process, a changed culture, and implementation of the principles of the MRP.

# Chapter 9

## Tips for success

> "'Come to the edge,' he said.
> They said, 'We are afraid.'
> 'Come to the edge,' he said.
> They came. He pushed them . . . and they flew."
> —Guillaume Appollinaire

This book was written to take some of the guesswork out of the various structures and processes behind shared governance. Throughout the chapters and sections, numerous strategies, case examples, and best practices have been provided to make the daily operations of shared governance meaningful and successful. This chapter lists additional tips and ideas to further entice you to enjoy the shared governance process and your journey in reshaping professional nursing practice for today and tomorrow.

## 22 tips for successful shared governance

1. Schedule a day-long retreat away from the organization to prepare organizational and nursing leaders to implement shared governance. If appropriate, discuss the role that shared governance plays in the ANCC Magnet Recognition Program® (MRP) journey. Have subject matter experts present topic discussions on specific points, such as leadership, shared governance partners, steering committee formation, design team for the shared governance model, a business case for shared governance, and new roles of staff nurses and the multidisciplinary team members.

2. **Create expectations for staff contributions, beginning in the new employee orientation and continuing throughout their careers.**

3. Communicate, communicate, communicate! Have a Nursing Town Hall meeting at least once per quarter to facilitate open communication among nursing staff and leaders.

4. **Administer the Index of Professional Nursing Governance surveys and see how your organization "measures up"—help build the repository of information on the efficacy and value of shared governance in healthcare settings.**

5. Visit the Online Journal of Issues in Nursing, Shared Governance edition © 2004 at *www.nursingworld.org/ojin/*.

6. **Use journal clubs, for example, to bring nursing research to the bedside and to engage staff nurses in evidence-based practice for developing and implementing advanced decision-making and critical thinking.**

7. Let staff nurses meet each year to review organizational competencies and unit/area needs and to determine which competencies they will focus on for that year (e.g., high-risk/time sensitive, changed, problematic, new).

8. **Train every registered nurse on each unit/area to be charge or lead nurse. Rotate the role and responsibilities to encourage leadership skills development and shared decision-making among all team members.**

9. Involve all staff members in preparing and adapting their schedules to accommodate the needs of their work area. Open staffing to flexible schedules and peer-negotiated days off. Nurse leaders should step in only if there are irreconcilable differences, if there are stalemates, or to help nurses with the process. Responsibility here, as in other areas of shared governance, must be coupled with appropriate levels of authority and accountability to be successful.

10. **Communicate the process, expectations, roles, and responsibilities for nurses engaged in shared decision-making throughout the organization, not just on their units/areas.**

11. Address management and leadership styles in the shared governance process model selected.

12. **Make sure that *all* nurse executives, directors, supervisors, and managers are trained and engaged in the shared governance process model development before bringing staff into the mix. Otherwise, the nursing leaders may become confused or uncomfortable and inadvertently sabotage the work before it even begins.**

13. Recognize and celebrate those staff nurses who represent their peers and patients on the shared governance councils and in the community. Support them through creative staffing, "surprise" celebrations, quiet encouragements, and provision of whatever resources they need to be successful.

14. **Prepare, support, and encourage nurse change champions to help lead strategic change and facilitate the implementation of shared governance.**

15. Display unit exhibits, bulletin boards, and other learning events; create staff activities; and hold staff celebrations/awards.

16. **Create an organizational "who's who" of your best practice nurses, MRP Champions (if applicable), and hospital heroes to share with the organization and community.**

17. Celebrate, celebrate, celebrate every milestone and moment of excellence completed along the way.

18. **Attend workshops and seminars on shared governance, MRP designation, and leadership in professional practice.**

19. Network with organizations that have implemented shared governance successfully or are just beginning their journey (such as those presented in this book). Share best practices with them.

20. **Once shared governance is fully implemented and the organizational culture is ready, consider beginning the MRP journey.**

21. *Many companies define Human Resources as being solely responsible for attraction, motivation, and retention. Our approach has always been to entrust our great [nurses] with that responsibility.* —Elizabeth Barrett

22. **Think about YOUR ideas for success in shared governance.**

## Conclusion

Shared governance is evidence that the organization supports and values the personal and professional development of all healthcare team members. Nurse leaders and staff nurses benefit when they emphasize providing in-depth, quality orientations for new employees and those who transition into new positions, as well as ongoing inservices and career development through shared decision-making.

Culture changes that reflect the continuous growth and maturity of professional nurses begin with the development of nurse leaders. What is true of safety in airplane flights is true of nursing leadership: Before you can help someone else, you have to put on your own oxygen mask first. Nursing executives and managers must first understand, embrace, and role-model shared governance through relational empowerment and servant leadership for it to be fully realized in their organization. Gear up, take a deep breath, and enjoy the journey!

# Bibliography

Allen, D., Calkin, J., and Peterson, M. (1988). "Making shared governance work: A conceptual model." *Journal of Nursing Administration,* 18(1), 37–43.

Alvarado, K., Boblin-Cummings, S., and Goddard, P. (2000). "Experiencing nursing governance: Developing a post merger nursing committee structure." *Canadian Journal of Nursing Leadership,* 13(4), 30–35.

American Association of Colleges of Nursing (2002). *AACN white paper: Hallmarks of the professional nursing practice environment.* Washington, DC.

American Hospital Association (2002). *How hospital leaders can build a thriving workforce.* Washington, DC: AHA Commission on Workforce for Hospitals and Health Systems.

American Nurses Association (2003). "ANA reorganizes structure to better meet nurses' needs." *The American Nurse,* 35(4), 1, 12–13.

American Organization of Nurse Executives (2000). *Perspectives on the nursing shortage: A blueprint for action.* Chicago.

Anderson, B. (1992). "Voyage to shared governance." *Nursing Management,* 23(11), 65–67.

Anderson, E. (2000). *Empowerment, job satisfaction, and professional governance of nurses in hospitals with and without shared governance.* Doctoral dissertation. School of Nursing, Louisiana State University Medical Center; New Orleans.

Anthony, M. K. (2004). "Shared governance models: The theory, practice, and evidence." *Online Journal of Issues in Nursing,* 9(1/4), *http://nursingworld.org/ojin/topic23/tpc23_4.htm.*

Arbinger Institute. (2002). *Leadership and self-deception: Getting out of the box.* San Francisco: Berrett-Koehler Publishers, Inc.

Barker, A. M., Sullivan, D. T., and Emery, M. J. (2006). *Leadership competencies for clinical managers: The renaissance of transformational leadership.* Sudbury, MA: Jones and Bartlett Publishers.

Benner, P. (1984). *From novice to expert: Excellence and power in clinical nursing practice.* Menlo Park, CA: Addison-Wesley Publishing Company.

Beyea, S. C., and Slattery, M. J. (2006). *Evidence-based practice in nursing: A guide to successful implementation.* Marblehead, MA: HCPro, Inc.

Black, J. S., and Gregersen, H. B. (2003). *Leading strategic change: Breaking through the brain barrier.* Upper Saddle River, NJ: Pearson Education, Inc.

Brennan, P. F., and Anthony, M. K. (2000). "Measuring nursing practice models using multi-attribute utility theory." *Research in Nursing and Health,* 23, 372–382.

Brooks, S.B., Olsen, P., Rieger-Kligys, S., and Mooney, L. (1995). "Peer review: An approach to performance evaluation in a professional practice model." *Critical Care Nursing Quarterly,* 18(3), 36–47.

Buckingham, M., and Coffman, C. (1999). *First, break all the rules: What the world's greatest managers do differently.* The Gallup Organization. New York: Simon and Schuster.

Cashman, K. (1998). *Leadership from the inside out: Becoming a leader for life.* Provo, UT: Executive Excellence Publishing.

Cottrell, D., and Adams, A. (2006). *The next level: Leading beyond the status quo.* Dallas: CornerStone Leadership Institute.

Covey, S. R. (1991). *Principle-centered leadership.* New York: Summit Books.

Daugherty, J., and Hart, P. (1993). "Shared governance." *Nursing Management,* 24(4), 100–101.

DeBaca, V., Jones, K., and Tornabeni, J. (1993). "A cost-benefit analysis of shared governance." *Journal of Nursing Administration,* 23(7/8), 50–57.

Evan, K., Aubry, K., Hawkins, M., Curley, T.A., and Porter-O'Grady, T. (1995). "Whole systems shared governance: A model for the integrated health system." *Journal of Nursing Administration,* 25(5), 18–27.

Farley, V. M. (2000). *Future tense, or . . . tense future.* Lincoln, NE: toExcel Publications.

Finkler, S.A., Kovner, C.T., Knickman, J.R., and Hendrickson, G. (1994). "Innovation in nursing: A benefit/cost analysis." *Nursing Economic$,* 12(1), 18–27.

Fournies, F. F. (1999). *Why employees don't do what they are supposed to do and what to do about it.* New York: McGraw-Hill.

Gardner, D., and Cummings, C. (1994). "Total quality management and shared governance: synergistic processes." *Nursing Administration Quarterly,* 18(4), 56–64.

George, V.M., Burke, L.J., and Rodgers, B.L. (1997). "Research-based planning for change: Assessing nurses' attitudes toward governance and professional practice autonomy after hospital acquisition." *Journal of Nursing Administration,* 27(5), 53–61.

Green, A., and Jordan, C. (2002). "Workplace advocacy and workplace issues." In B. Cherry and S. Jacob (Eds.), *Contemporary nursing: Issues, trends, and management.* St. Louis: Mosby.

Green, A., and Jordan, C. (2004). "Common denominators: shared governance and work place advocacy—strategies for nurses to gain control over their practice." *Online Journal of Issues in Nursing,* 6(1/6), *http://nursingworld.org/ojin/topic23/tpc23_6.htm.*

Grote, D. (1995). *Discipline without punishment: The proven strategy that turns problem employees into superior performers.* New York: AMACOM, a division of American Management Association.

Harvey, E., and Lucia, A. (1995). *Walk the talk . . . and get the results you want.* Foreword by Kenneth H. Blanchard. Dallas: Performance Publishing Company.

Havens, D. S., and Aiken, L. H. (February 1999). "Shaping systems to promote desired outcomes: The Magnet hospital model." *Journal of Nursing Administration,* 29, 14–20.

Hess, R. G. (2004). "From bedside to boardroom—nursing shared governance." *Online Journal of Issues in Nursing,* 9(1). Accessed June 2, 2006, online at *www.nursingworld.org/ojin/topic23/tpc23_1.htm.*

Hess, R. G. (1995). "Shared governance: Nursing's 20th century tower of Babel." *Journal of Nursing Administration,* 25(5).

Hess, R.G. (1996). "Measuring shared governance outcomes." *Nursing Economic$,* 14(4), 254.

Hess, R.G. (1998). "Measuring nursing governance." *Nursing Research,* 47(1), 35–42.

Hess, R. (1998). "A breed apart—real shared governance." *Journal of Shared Governance,* 4(3): 5–6.

Hoffart, N., and Woods, C. (1996). "Elements of a nursing professional practice model." *Journal of Professional Nursing,* 12(6), 354–364.

Howell, J., Frederick, J., Ollinger, B., Hess, R., et al. (2001). "Can nurses govern in a government agency?" *Journal of Nursing Administration,* 31: 187–195.

Kohn, Corrigan and Donaldson (Eds.) (1999). *To err is human: Building a safer health system.* Institute of Medicine, Committee on Quality Health Care in America. Washington, DC: National Academy Press.

Ireson, C., and McGillis, G. (1998). "A multidisciplinary shared governance model." *Nursing Management,* 29(2), 37–39.

Jacoby, J., and Terpstra, M. (1990). "Collaborative governance: Model for professional autonomy." *Nursing Management,* 21(2), 42–44.

Jenkins, J. (1988). "A nursing governance and practice model: What are the costs?" *Nursing Economic$,* 6(6), 302–311.

Jones, G. (2004). *Organizational theory, design, and change (4th ed.).* Upper Saddle River, NJ: Pearson, Prentice Hall.

Jones, C. B., Stasiowski, S., Simons, B. J., Boyd, N. J., and Lucas, M.D. (1993). "Shared governance and the nursing practice environment." *Nursing Economic$,* 11, 208–214.

Jones, L. S., and Ortiz, M. (1989). "Increasing nursing autonomy and recognition through shared governance." *Nursing Administration Quarterly,* 13(4), 11–16.

Koloroutis, M. (Ed.) (2004). *Relationship-based care: A model for transforming practice.* Minneapolis: Creative Health Care Management.

Kovner, C.T., Hendrickson, G., Knickman, J.R., and Finkler, S.A. (1993). "Changing the delivery of nursing care: Implementation issues and qualitative findings." *Journal of Nursing Administration,* 23(11), 24–34.

Laschinger, H.K.S., Almost, J., and Tuer-Hodes, D. (2003). "Workplace empowerment and magnet hospital characteristics." *Journal of Nursing Administration,* 33(7/8), 410–422.

Laschinger, H.K.S., and Havens, D.S. (1996). "Staff nurse empowerment and perceived control over nursing practice." *Journal of Nursing Administration,* 26(9), 27–35.

Laschinger, H.K.S., Sabiston, J.A., and Kutszcher, L. (1997). "Empowerment and staff nurse decision involvement in nursing work environment: Testing Kanter's theory of structural power in organizations." *Research in Nursing and Health,* 20, 341–352.

Laschinger, H.K.S., Wong, C., McMahon, L., and Kaufman, C. (1999). "Leader behavior impact on staff nurse empowerment, job tension, and work effectiveness." *Journal of Nursing Administration,* 29(5), 28–39.

Ludemann, R.S., and Brown, C. (1989). "Staff perceptions of shared governance." *Nursing Administration Quarterly,* 13(4), 49–56.

Maas, M., and Jacox, A. (1977). *Guidelines for Nurse Autonomy/Patient Welfare.* New York: Appelton-Century-Crofts.

Mallik, M., and Raffert, A. (2000). "Diffusion of the concept of patient advocacy." *Journal of Nursing Scholarship,* 32(4), 399–404.

Maxwell, J. C. (2006). *The INJOY Group: EQUIP™—Affecting leadership development in emerging countries, American urban centers, and academic communities.* Online at *www.INJOY.com.*

Maxwell, J. C. (2001). *The 17 indisputable laws of teamwork: Embrace them and empower your team.* Nashville: Thomas Nelson Publishers.

Maxwell, J. C. (1999). *The 21 indisputable qualities of a leader: Becoming the person others will want to follow.* Nashville,: Thomas Nelson Publishers.

Maxwell, J. C. (1998). *The 21 indisputable laws of leadership: Follow them and people will follow you.* Nashville: Thomas Nelson Publishers.

Maxwell, J. C. (1993). *The winning attitude.* Nashville: Thomas Nelson Publishers.

McClure, M. L., and Hinshaw, A. S. (Eds.) (2002). *Magnet hospitals revisited.* American Academy of Nursing. Washington, DC: American Nurses Publishing.

McDonagh, K., Rhodes, B., Sharkey, K., and Goodroe, J. (1989). "Shared governance at Saint Joseph's hospital of Atlanta: A mature professional practice model." *Nursing Administration Quarterly*, 13(4), 17–28.

Merton, R. (1960). "The search for professional status." *American Journal of Nursing*, 60, 662–664.

Metcalf, R., and Tate, R. (1995). "Shared governance in the endoscopy department." *Gastroenterology Nursing*, 18(3), 96–99.

Minnen, T., Berger, E., Ames, A., Dubree, M., Baker, W., and Spinella, J. (1993). "Sustaining work redesign innovations through shared governance." *Journal of Nursing Administration*, 23 (7/8), 35–40.

National Press Publications (Ed.). (2001). *The manager's role as coach: Motivate, mentor and coach your most valuable asset—your people— to achieve professional excellence* (2nd ed). Shawnee Mission, KS: National Press Publications, Inc.

Nightingale, F. (1992). *Notes on nursing: What it is, and what it is not.* Philadelphia: Lippincott Williams and Wilkins.

Nursing Executive Center Practice Brief (2005). *Toward Staff-Driven Decision Making. Assessing, Building, and Sustaining a Shared Governance Model.* Washington, DC: The Advisory Board Company. Entire IPNG included.

O'May, F., and Buchan, J. (1999). "Shared governance: A literature review." *International Journal of Nursing Studies*, 36, 281–300.

Ortiz, M.E., Gehring, P., Sovie, M.D. (1987). "Moving to shared governance." *American Journal of Nursing,* 87(7), 923–926.

Oster, M. J. (1991). *Vision-driven leadership.* Foreword by Kenneth H. Blanchard. San Bernardino, CA: Here's Life Publishers, Inc.

Page, A. (Ed.) (2004). *Keeping patients safe: Transforming the work environment of nurses.* Committee on the Work Environment for Nurses and Patient Safety, Board on Health Care Services, Institute of Medicine of the National Academies. Washington, DC: National Academy Press.

Perley, M. J., and Raab, A. (1994). "Beyond shared governance: Restructuring care delivery for self–managing work teams." *Nursing Administration Quarterly,* 19(1), 12–20.

Peters, T. J., and Waterman, Jr., R. H. (1982). *In search of excellence: Lessons from America's best-run companies.* New York: Warner Books.

Peterson, M.E., and Allen, D.G. (1986a). "Shared governance: A strategy for transforming organizations, Part 1." *Journal of Nursing Administration,* 16(1), 9–12.

Peterson, M.E., and Allen, D.G. (1986b). "Shared governance: A strategy for transforming organizations, Part 2." *Journal of Nursing Administration,* 16(2), 11–16.

Pettitt, L. (2002). "Nursing governance and staff nurses self-concept." Master's thesis. Gardner-Webb University; Boiling Springs, NC.

Porter-O'Grady, T. (1987). "Shared governance and new organizational models." *Nursing Economic$,* 5(6), 281–286.

Porter-O'Grady, T. (1989). "Shared governance: Reality or sham?" *American Journal of Nursing Administration,* 89(3), 350–351.

Porter-O'Grady, T. (1990). *Reorganization of nursing practice: Creating the corporate venture.* Rockville, MD: Aspen Publications.

Porter-O'Grady, T. (1991). "Shared governance for nursing part II: Putting the organization into action." *AORN Journal,* 53(3), 694–703.

Porter-O'Grady, T. (1992). *Implementing shared governance: Creating a professional organization.* St. Louis, MO: Mosby-Year Books.

Porter-O'Grady, T. (1995). Letter to the editor. *Journal of Nursing Administration,* 25(7/8), 8–9.

Porter-O'Grady, T (1996). "More thoughts on shared governance." *Nursing Economic$,* 14(4), 254–255.

Porter-O'Grady, T. (2001). "Is shared governance still relevant?" *Journal of Nursing Administration,* 31(10), 468–473.

Porter-O'Grady, T. (2002). "Nurses as partners." *Hospitals and Health Networks/AHA,* 76(12), 10, 12.

Porter-O'Grady, T. (2003a). "A different age for leadership, Part 1: New context, new content." *Journal of Nursing Administration,* 33(2), 105–110.

Porter-O'Grady, T. (2003b). "A different age for leadership, Part 2: New rules, new roles." *Journal of Nursing Administration,* 33(3), 173–178.

Porter-O'Grady, T. (2003c). "Researching shared governance: A futility of focus." *Journal of Nursing Administration,* 33(4), 251–252.

Porter-O'Grady, T. (2004). Shared governance implementation manual. Atlanta: Tim Porter-O'Grady Associates, Inc.

Porter-O'Grady, T., and Finnigan, S. (1984). *Shared governance for nursing: A creative approach to professional accountability.* Rockville, MD: Aspen Systems Corp.

Porter-O'Grady, T., and Hitchings, K. S. (November 8, 2005). *Shared governance: How to create and sustain a culture of nurse empowerment.* Audioconference. Marblehead, MA: HCPro, Inc.

Porter-O'Grady, T., Hawkins, M. A., and Parker, M. L. (Eds.). (1997). *Whole-systems shared governance: Architecture for integration.* Gaithersburg, MD: Aspen Publishers.

Prince, S.B. (1997). "Shared governance: Sharing power and opportunity." *Journal of Nursing Administration,* 27(3), 28–35.

Relf, M. (1995). "Increasing job satisfaction and motivation while reducing nursing turnover though the implementation of shared governance." *Critical Care Nursing Quarterly,* 18(3), 7–13.

Richards, K.C., Ragland, P., Zehler, J., Dotson, K., Berube, M., Tygart, M.W., et al. (1999). "Implementing a councilor model: Process and outcomes." *Journal of Nursing Administration,* 29(7/8), 19–27.

Rose, M., and Reynolds, B. (1995). "How to make professional practice models work." *Critical Care Nursing Quarterly,* 18(3), 106.

Sabiston, J.A., and Lashinger, H.K.S. (1995). "Staff nurse work empowerment and perceived autonomy." *Journal of Nursing Administration,* 25(9), 42–50.

Senge, P., Kleiner, A., Roberts, C., Ross, R. B., and Smith, B. J. (1994). *The fifth discipline fieldbook: Strategies and tools for building a learning organization.* New York: Doubleday.

Shidler, H., Pencak, M., and McFolling, S.D. (1989). "Professional nursing staff: A model of self–governance for nursing." *Nursing Administration Quarterly,* 13(4), 1–9.

Song, R., Daly, B.J., Rudy, E.B., Douglas, S., and Dyer, M.A. (1997). "Nurses' job satisfaction, absenteeism, and turnover after implementing a special care unit practice model." *Research in Nursing and Health,* 20, 443–452.

Staff. (1996). Interview of Robert Hess and Tim Porter-O'Grady addressing 13 questions concerning the progress and future of shared governance. *Journal of Shared Governance,* 2(4):11–15.

Stumpf, L.R. (2001). "A comparison of governance types and patient satisfaction outcomes." *Journal of Nursing Administration,* 31(4), 196–202.

Thrasher, T., Bossman, V.M., Carroll, S., Cook, B., Cherry, K., Kopras, S.M, et al. (1992). "Empowering the clinical nurse through quality assurance in a shared governance setting." *Journal of Nursing Care Quarterly,* 6(2), 15–19.

Turkel, M. C. (2004). *HCPro's Guide to Assessing, Pursuing, and Achieving Excellence in the ANCC Magnet Recognition Program*. Marblehead, MA: HCPro, Inc.

Upenieks, V. V. (September 2003). "What constitutes effective leadership? Perceptions of Magnet and nonMagnet nurse leaders." *The Journal of Nursing Administration,* 33, 456–467.

Vilardo, L.E. (1993). "Linking collaborative governance with job satisfaction." *Nursing Management,* 24, 75.

Weinberg, D. B. (2003). "Code green: Money-driven hospitals and the dismantling of nursing." Ithaca, NY: Cornell University Press.

Westrope, R.A., Vaughn, L., Bott, M., and Taunton, R.L. (1995). "Shared governance: From vision to reality." *Journal of Nursing Administration,* 25(12), 45–54.

Wright, D. (2002). "R+A+A: The secret formula for making communication and delegation easier." Video 4 in the *Moments of Excellence* video series. Minneapolis: Creative Health Care Management.

Zelauskas, B., and Howes, D.G. (1992). "The effects of implementing a professional practice model." *Journal of Nursing Administration,* 22(7/8), 18–23.

# Appendix A

## Index of Professional Nursing Governance

# PROFESSIONAL NURSING GOVERNANCE

*Please provide the following information. The information you provide is IMPORTANT. Please be sure to complete ALL questions. Remember confidentiality will be maintained at all times.* Today's Date _____

1. Sex: _____ Male _____ Female      2. Age: _____

3. Please indicate your BASIC nursing educational preparation:

_____ Nursing Diploma

_____ Associate Degree in Nursing

_____ Baccalaureate Degree in Nursing

4. Please indicate the HIGHEST educational degree that you have attained at this point in time:

_____ Nursing Diploma

_____ Associate Degree in Nursing

_____ Baccalaureate Degree in Nursing

_____ Master's Degree in Nursing, Specialty

_____ Master's Degree, Non-nursing

_____ Doctorate, Nursing

_____ Doctorate, Non-nursing

5. Employment Status:

_____ Full-time, 36-40 hours per week

_____ Part-time, less than 36 hours per week

6. Please specify the number of years that you have been practicing nursing (specify number of hours/week): _____

7. Please indicate the title of your present position _____

8. Please indicate the type of nursing unit that you work on:

_____ Medical

_____ Surgical

_____ Critical Care

_____ Operating Room

_____ Recovery Room

_____ Emergency Room

_____ Clinic

_____ Maternity

_____ Pediatrics

_____ Psychiatry

_____ Education

_____ Quality Management

_____ Outside Nursing

_____ Other (please specify): _____

9. Please specify the number of years you have worked in this institution _____

10. Please specify the number of years you have been in this present position _____

11. Have you received any specialty certifications from professional organizations?
_____ Yes _____ No
If YES, please specify the type of certification and year received _____

---

*In your hospital, please circle the group that CONTROLS the following areas:*

1 = Nursing management/administration only
2 = Primarily nursing management/administration with some staff nurse input
3 = Equally shared by staff nurses and nursing management/administration
4 = Primarily staff nurses with some nursing management/administration input
5 = Staff nurses only

## PART 1

| | | |
|---|---|---|
| 1. Determining what activities nurses can do at the bedside. | | 1 2 3 4 5 |
| 2. Developing and evaluating patient care standards and quality assurance/improvement activities. | | 1 2 3 4 5 |
| 3. Setting levels of qualifications for nursing positions. | | 1 2 3 4 5 |
| 4. Evaluating (performance appraisals) nursing personnel. | | 1 2 3 4 5 |
| 5. Determining activities of ancillary nursing personnel (aides, unit clerks, etc.). | | 1 2 3 4 5 |
| 6. Conducting disciplinary action of nursing personnel. | | 1 2 3 4 5 |
| 7. Assessing and providing for the professional/educational development of the nursing staff. | | 1 2 3 4 5 |
| 8. Making hiring decisions about RNs and their nursing staff. | | 1 2 3 4 5 |
| 9. Promoting RNs and other nursing staff. | | 1 2 3 4 5 |
| 10. Appointing nursing personnel to management and leadership positions. | | 1 2 3 4 5 |
| 11. Selecting products used in nursing care. | | 1 2 3 4 5 |
| 12. Incorporating research ideas into nursing care. | | 1 2 3 4 5 |
| 13. Determining methods of nursing care delivery (e.g. primary, team, case management). | | 1 2 3 4 5 |

# PROFESSIONAL NURSING GOVERNANCE

*In your hospital, please circle the group that INFLUENCES the following activities:*

1 = Nursing management/administration only
2 = Primarily nursing management/administration with some staff nurse input
3 = Equally shared by staff nurses and nursing management/administration
4 = Primarily staff nurses with some nursing management/administration input
5 = Staff nurses only

## PART II

| | 1 | 2 | 3 | 4 | 5 |
|---|---|---|---|---|---|
| 14. Determining how many and what level of nursing staff is needed for routine patient care. | 1 | 2 | 3 | 4 | 5 |
| 15. Adjusting staffing levels to meet fluctuations in patient census and acuity. | 1 | 2 | 3 | 4 | 5 |
| 16. Making daily patient care assignments for nursing personnel. | 1 | 2 | 3 | 4 | 5 |
| 17. Monitoring and procuring supplies for nursing care and support functions. | 1 | 2 | 3 | 4 | 5 |
| 18. Regulating the flow of patient admissions, transfers, and discharges. | 1 | 2 | 3 | 4 | 5 |
| 19. Formulating annual unit budgets for personnel, supplies, equipment and education. | 1 | 2 | 3 | 4 | 5 |
| 20. Recommending nursing salaries, raises and benefits. | 1 | 2 | 3 | 4 | 5 |
| 21. Consulting nursing services outside of the unit (e.g. administration, psychiatric, medical-surgical). | 1 | 2 | 3 | 4 | 5 |
| 22. Consulting hospital services outside of nursing (e.g. dietary, social service, pharmacy, human resources, finance). | 1 | 2 | 3 | 4 | 5 |
| 23. Making recommendations concerning other departments' resources. | 1 | 2 | 3 | 4 | 5 |
| 24. Determining cost effective measures such as patient placement and referrals (e.g. placement of ventilator-dependent patients, early discharge of patients to home health care). | 1 | 2 | 3 | 4 | 5 |
| 25. Recommending new hospital services or specialties (e.g. gerontology, mental health, birthing centers). | 1 | 2 | 3 | 4 | 5 |
| 26. Creating new clinical positions. | 1 | 2 | 3 | 4 | 5 |
| 27. Creating new administrative or support positions. | 1 | 2 | 3 | 4 | 5 |

*According to the following indicators in your hospital, please circle which group has OFFICIAL AUTHORITY (i.e. authority granted and recognized by the hospital) to control practice and influence the resources that support it:*

1 = Nursing management/administration only
2 = Primarily nursing management/administration with some staff nurse input
3 = Equally shared by staff nurses and nursing management/administration
4 = Primarily staff nurses with some nursing management/administration input
5 = Staff nurses only

## PART III

| | 1 | 2 | 3 | 4 | 5 |
|---|---|---|---|---|---|
| 28. Written policies and procedures that state what nurses can do in direct patient care. | 1 | 2 | 3 | 4 | 5 |
| 29. Written patient care standards and quality assurance/improvement programs. | 1 | 2 | 3 | 4 | 5 |
| 30. Mandatory RN credentialing levels (licensure, education, certifications) for hiring, continued employment, promotions and raises. | 1 | 2 | 3 | 4 | 5 |
| 31. Written process for evaluating nursing personnel (performance appraisal). | 1 | 2 | 3 | 4 | 5 |
| 32. Organizational charts that show job titles and who reports to whom. | 1 | 2 | 3 | 4 | 5 |
| 33. Written guidelines for disciplining nursing personnel. | 1 | 2 | 3 | 4 | 5 |
| 34. Annual requirements for continuing inservices. | 1 | 2 | 3 | 4 | 5 |
| 35. Procedures for hiring and transferring nursing personnel. | 1 | 2 | 3 | 4 | 5 |
| 36. Policies regulating promotion of nursing personnel to management and leadership positions. | 1 | 2 | 3 | 4 | 5 |
| 37. Procedures for generating schedules for RNs and other nursing staff. | 1 | 2 | 3 | 4 | 5 |

# PROFESSIONAL NURSING GOVERNANCE

*In your hospital, please circle the group that PARTICIPATES in the following activities:*

1 = Nursing management/administration only
2 = Primarily nursing management/administration with some staff nurse input
3 = Equally shared by staff nurses and nursing management/administration
4 = Primarily staff nurses with some nursing management/administration input
5 = Staff nurses only

| | | | | | |
|---|---|---|---|---|---|
| 38. Acuity and patient classification systems for determining how many and what level of nursing staff is needed for routine patient care. | 1 | 2 | 3 | 4 | 5 |
| 39. Mechanisms for determining staffing levels when there are fluctuations in patient census and acuity. | 1 | 2 | 3 | 4 | 5 |
| 40. Procedures for determining daily patient care assignments. | 1 | 2 | 3 | 4 | 5 |
| 41. Daily methods for monitoring and obtaining supplies for nursing care and support functions. | 1 | 2 | 3 | 4 | 5 |
| 42. Procedures for controlling the flow of patient admissions, transfers and discharges. | 1 | 2 | 3 | 4 | 5 |
| 43. Process for recommending and formulating annual unit budgets for personnel, supplies, major equipment and education. | 1 | 2 | 3 | 4 | 5 |
| 44. Procedures for adjusting nursing salaries, raises and benefits. | 1 | 2 | 3 | 4 | 5 |
| 45. Formal mechanisms for consulting and enlisting the support of nursing services outside of the unit (e.g. administration, psychiatric, medical-surgical). | 1 | 2 | 3 | 4 | 5 |
| 46. Formal mechanisms for consulting and enlisting the support of hospital service outside of nursing (e.g. dietary, social service, pharmacy, physical therapy). | 1 | 2 | 3 | 4 | 5 |
| 47. Procedure for restricting or limiting patient care (e.g. closing hospital beds, going on ER bypass). | 1 | 2 | 3 | 4 | 5 |
| 48. Location of and access to office space. | 1 | 2 | 3 | 4 | 5 |
| 49. Access to office equipment (e.g. phones, personal computers, copy machines). | 1 | 2 | 3 | 4 | 5 |

## PART IV

| | | | | | |
|---|---|---|---|---|---|
| 50. Participation in unit committees for clinical practice. | 1 | 2 | 3 | 4 | 5 |
| 51. Participation in unit committees for administrative matters such as staffing, scheduling and budgeting. | 1 | 2 | 3 | 4 | 5 |
| 52. Participation in nursing departmental committees for clinical practice. | 1 | 2 | 3 | 4 | 5 |
| 53. Participation in nursing departmental committees for administrative matters such as staffing, scheduling, and budgeting. | 1 | 2 | 3 | 4 | 5 |
| 54. Participation in multidisciplinary professional committees (physicians, other hospital professions and departments) for collaborative practice. | 1 | 2 | 3 | 4 | 5 |
| 55. Participation in hospital administration committees for matters such as employee benefits and strategic planning. | 1 | 2 | 3 | 4 | 5 |
| 56. Forming new unit committees. | 1 | 2 | 3 | 4 | 5 |
| 57. Forming new nursing departmental committees. | 1 | 2 | 3 | 4 | 5 |
| 58. Forming new multidisciplinary professional committees. | 1 | 2 | 3 | 4 | 5 |
| 59. Forming new hospital administration committees. | 1 | 2 | 3 | 4 | 5 |

# PROFESSIONAL NURSING GOVERNANCE

*In your hospital, please circle the group that has ACCESS TO INFORMATION about the following activities:*

1 = Nursing management/administration only
2 = Primarily nursing management/administration with some staff nurse input
3 = Equally shared by staff nurses and nursing management/administration
4 = Primarily staff nurses with some nursing management/administration input
5 = Staff nurses only

## PART V

60. The quality of hospital nursing practice. 1 2 3 4 5
61. Compliance of hospital nursing practice with requirements of surveying agencies (Joint Commission, state and federal government, professional groups). 1 2 3 4 5
62. Unit's projected budget and actual expenses. 1 2 3 4 5
63. Hospital's financial status. 1 2 3 4 5
64. Unit and nursing departmental goals and objectives for this year. 1 2 3 4 5
65. Hospital's strategic plans for the next few years. 1 2 3 4 5
66. Results of patient satisfaction surveys. 1 2 3 4 5
67. Physician/nurse satisfaction with their collaborative practice. 1 2 3 4 5
68. Current hospital status of nurse turnover and vacancies. 1 2 3 4 5
69. Nurses' satisfaction with their general practice. 1 2 3 4 5
70. Nurses' satisfaction with their salaries and benefits. 1 2 3 4 5
71. Management's opinion of bedside nursing practice. 1 2 3 4 5
72. Physicians' opinion of bedside nursing practice. 1 2 3 4 5
73. Nursing peers' opinion of bedside nursing practice. 1 2 3 4 5
74. Access to resources concerning recent advances in nursing practice (e.g.journals and books, library). 1 2 3 4 5

*In your hospital, please circle the group that has the ABILITY to:*

1 = Nursing management/administration only
2 = Primarily nursing management/administration with some staff nurse input
3 = Equally shared by staff nurses and nursing management/administration
4 = Primarily staff nurses with some nursing management/administration input
5 = Staff nurses only

## PART VI

75. Negotiate solutions to conflicts among professional nurses. 1 2 3 4 5
76. Negotiate solutions to conflicts between professional nurses and physicians. 1 2 3 4 5
77. Negotiate solutions to conflicts between professional nurses and other hospital services (respiratory, dietary, etc). 1 2 3 4 5
78. Negotiate solutions to conflicts between professional nurses and nursing management. 1 2 3 4 5
79. Negotiate solutions to conflicts between professional nurses and hospital administration. 1 2 3 4 5
80. Create a formal grievance procedure. 1 2 3 4 5
81. Write the goals and objectives of a nursing unit. 1 2 3 4 5
82. Write the philosophy, goals and objectives of the nursing department. 1 2 3 4 5
83. Formulate the mission, philosophy, goals and objectives of the hospital. 1 2 3 4 5
84. Write unit policies and procedures. 1 2 3 4 5
85. Determine nursing departmental policies and procedures. 1 2 3 4 5
86. Determine hospital-wide policies and procedures. 1 2 3 4 5

# Appendix B

## Index of Professional Governance

# PROFESSIONAL GOVERNANCE

Please provide the following information. The information you provide is IMPORTANT. Please be sure to complete ALL questions. Remember confidentiality will be maintained at all times.    Today's Date _____

1. Sex: _____ Male _____ Female    2. Age: _____

3. Please indicate your profession:
   _____ Accountant          _____ Physician
   _____ Dietician           _____ Registered Nurse
   _____ Pharmacist          _____ Respiratory Therapist
   _____ Physical Therapist  _____ Social Worker
   _____ Other

4. Please indicate your HIGHEST educational degree:
   _____ Diploma             _____ Master's Degree
   _____ Associate Degree    _____ Doctorate
   _____ Baccalaureate Degree

5. Employment Status:
   _____ Full-time, 36-40 hours per week
   _____ Part-time, less than 36 hours per week (specify number of hours/week): _____

6. Please specify the number of years that you have been practicing _____

7. Please indicate the title of your present position _____

8. Please indicate your clinical specialty:
   _____ Medical/Surgical    _____ Maternity
   _____ Critical Care       _____ Pediatrics
   _____ Operating Room      _____ Psychiatry
   _____ Recovery Room       _____ Education
   _____ Emergency Room      _____ Quality Management
   _____ Clinic              _____ Case Management
   _____ Rehabilitation      _____ Other
                                   (please specify): _____

9. Please specify the number of years you have worked in this organization _____

10. Please specify the number of years you have been in your present position _____

11. Please rate your overall satisfaction with your professional practice within the organization (1 = lowest, 5 = highest):    1    2    3    4    5

---

In your hospital, please circle the group that CONTROLS the following areas:

1 = Management/administration only
2 = Primarily management/administration with some staff input
3 = Equally shared by staff and management/administration
4 = Primarily staff with some management/administration input
5 = Staff only

## PART I

1. Determining what activities your professional colleagues can do in their daily practice.    1    2    3    4    5

2. Developing and evaluating service standards and quality assurance/improvement activities.    1    2    3    4    5

3. Setting levels of qualifications for positions within your own discipline.    1    2    3    4    5

4. Evaluating (performance appraisals) professional personnel within your own discipline.    1    2    3    4    5

5. Determining activities of ancillary personnel (aides, clerks, secretaries, assistants, etc.).    1    2    3    4    5

6. Conducting disciplinary actions of colleagues within your discipline.    1    2    3    4    5

7. Assessing and providing for the professional/ educational development of professionals within your own discipline.    1    2    3    4    5

8. Making hiring decisions about professionals within your discipline and their support staff.    1    2    3    4    5

9. Promoting colleagues and their support staff.    1    2    3    4    5

10. Appointing personnel to management and leadership positions.    1    2    3    4    5

11. Selecting products used in your professional practice.    1    2    3    4    5

12. Incorporating research ideas into your professional practice.    1    2    3    4    5

13. Determining methods or systems for accomplishing the work of your discipline.    1    2    3    4    5

© 1998 Robert G. Hess, Jr., RN, PhD. To obtain permission for use, call (856)424-4270 or e-mail bobhess@voicenet.com. Printed with permission.

# PROFESSIONAL GOVERNANCE

*In your hospital, please circle the group that INFLUENCES the following activities:*

1 = Management/administration only
2 = Primarily management/administration with some staff input
3 = Equally shared by staff and management/administration
4 = Primarily staff with some management/administration input
5 = Staff only

## PART II

| | 1 | 2 | 3 | 4 | 5 |
|---|---|---|---|---|---|
| 14. Determining how many staff and what level of expertise is needed for routine work. | 1 | 2 | 3 | 4 | 5 |
| 15. Adjusting staffing levels to meet fluctuations in work demands. | 1 | 2 | 3 | 4 | 5 |
| 16. Making work assignments for professional and support staff. | 1 | 2 | 3 | 4 | 5 |
| 17. Monitoring and procuring supplies necessary for professional practice and support functions. | 1 | 2 | 3 | 4 | 5 |
| 18. Regulating the flow of services or patients/clients within the organization. | 1 | 2 | 3 | 4 | 5 |
| 19. Formulating annual unit budgets for personnel, supplies, equipment, and education for your own unit or work group. | 1 | 2 | 3 | 4 | 5 |
| 20. Recommending salaries, raises and benefits. | 1 | 2 | 3 | 4 | 5 |
| 21. Consulting services outside of your own unit or work group. | 1 | 2 | 3 | 4 | 5 |
| 22. Consulting hospital services outside of your own discipline. | 1 | 2 | 3 | 4 | 5 |
| 23. Making recommendations concerning other departments' resources. | 1 | 2 | 3 | 4 | 5 |
| 24. Determining cost-effective measures for professional practice. | 1 | 2 | 3 | 4 | 5 |
| 25. Recommending new services or ventures. | 1 | 2 | 3 | 4 | 5 |
| 26. Creating new clinical positions. | 1 | 2 | 3 | 4 | 5 |
| 27. Creating new administrative or support positions. | 1 | 2 | 3 | 4 | 5 |

*According to the following indicators in your hospital, please circle which group has OFFICIAL AUTHORITY (i.e. authority granted and recognized by the hospital) to control practice and influence the resources that support it:*

1 = Management/administration only
2 = Primarily management/administration with some staff input
3 = Equally shared by staff and management/administration
4 = Primarily staff with some management/administration input
5 = Staff only

## PART III

| | 1 | 2 | 3 | 4 | 5 |
|---|---|---|---|---|---|
| 28. Written policies and procedures that state what activities professional colleagues can do in their daily practice. | 1 | 2 | 3 | 4 | 5 |
| 29. Written service standards and quality improvement activities. | 1 | 2 | 3 | 4 | 5 |
| 30. Mandatory credentialing levels of professionals (licensure, education, certifications) for hiring, continued employment, promotions, and raises. | 1 | 2 | 3 | 4 | 5 |
| 31. Written process for evaluating professional personnel within your own discipline. | 1 | 2 | 3 | 4 | 5 |
| 32. Organizational charts that show job titles and who reports to whom. | 1 | 2 | 3 | 4 | 5 |
| 33. Written guidelines for disciplining personnel. | 1 | 2 | 3 | 4 | 5 |
| 34. Annual requirements for continuing education. | 1 | 2 | 3 | 4 | 5 |
| 35. Procedures for hiring and transferring personnel. | 1 | 2 | 3 | 4 | 5 |
| 36. Policies regulating promotion of professional personnel to management and leadership positions. | 1 | 2 | 3 | 4 | 5 |
| 37. Procedures for generating schedules for professionals within your own discipline and their support staff. | 1 | 2 | 3 | 4 | 5 |

# PROFESSIONAL GOVERNANCE

*In your hospital, please circle the group that PARTICIPATES in the following activities:*

1 = Management/administration only
2 = Primarily management/administration with some staff input
3 = Equally shared by staff and management/administration
4 = Primarily staff with some management/administration input
5 = Staff only

|  |  | | | | | |
|---|------|---|---|---|---|---|
| 38. | Systems for determining how many staff and what level of expertise is needed for the day-to-day work of your unit or work group. | 1 | 2 | 3 | 4 | 5 |
| 39. | Mechanisms for determining staffing levels when there are fluctuations in work demands. | 1 | 2 | 3 | 4 | 5 |
| 40. | Procedures for determining work assignments. | 1 | 2 | 3 | 4 | 5 |
| 41. | Daily methods for monitoring and obtaining supplies that support the practice of your professional group within the organization. | 1 | 2 | 3 | 4 | 5 |
| 42. | Procedures for controlling the flow of services and patients/clients within the organization. | 1 | 2 | 3 | 4 | 5 |
| 43. | Process for recommending and formulating annual budgets for personnel, supplies, equipment, and education for your own work group. | 1 | 2 | 3 | 4 | 5 |
| 44. | Procedures for adjusting professional personnel's salaries, raises, and benefits. | 1 | 2 | 3 | 4 | 5 |
| 45. | Formal mechanisms for consulting and enlisting the support of other professionals within your discipline who work outside of your work group. | 1 | 2 | 3 | 4 | 5 |
| 46. | Formal mechanisms for consulting and enlisting support of organizational services outside of your work group. | 1 | 2 | 3 | 4 | 5 |
| 47. | Procedure for restricting or limiting the amount of work you do. | 1 | 2 | 3 | 4 | 5 |
| 48. | Location of and access to office space. | 1 | 2 | 3 | 4 | 5 |
| 49. | Access to office equipment (e.g. phones, personal computers, copy machines). | 1 | 2 | 3 | 4 | 5 |

## PART IV

|  |  | | | | | |
|---|------|---|---|---|---|---|
| 50. | Unit or work-group committees that deal with professional practice. | 1 | 2 | 3 | 4 | 5 |
| 51. | Unit or work-group committees that deal with administrative matters such as staffing, scheduling and budgeting. | 1 | 2 | 3 | 4 | 5 |
| 52. | Departmental committees that deal with professional practice. | 1 | 2 | 3 | 4 | 5 |
| 53. | Departmental committees that deal with administrative matters such as staffing, scheduling, and budgeting. | 1 | 2 | 3 | 4 | 5 |
| 54. | Multidisciplinary professional committees for collaborative practice. | 1 | 2 | 3 | 4 | 5 |
| 55. | Organizational administrative committees for matters such as employee benefits and strategic planning. | 1 | 2 | 3 | 4 | 5 |
| 56. | Formation of new unit or work-group committees. | 1 | 2 | 3 | 4 | 5 |
| 57. | Formation of new departmental committees within your own discipline. | 1 | 2 | 3 | 4 | 5 |
| 58. | Formation of new multidisciplinary professional committees. | 1 | 2 | 3 | 4 | 5 |
| 59. | Formation of new organizational administration committees. | 1 | 2 | 3 | 4 | 5 |

# PROFESSIONAL GOVERNANCE

*In your hospital, please circle the group that has ACCESS TO INFORMATION about the following activities:*

1 = Management/administration only
2 = Primarily management/administration with some staff input
3 = Equally shared by staff and management/administration
4 = Primarily staff with some management/administration input
5 = Staff only

## PART V

| | 1 | 2 | 3 | 4 | 5 |
|---|---|---|---|---|---|
| 60. Quality of professional practice. | 1 | 2 | 3 | 4 | 5 |
| 61. Compliance of your organization with requirements of surveying agencies (e.g. JCAHO, state and federal government, professional groups). | 1 | 2 | 3 | 4 | 5 |
| 62. Your work group's projected budget and actual expenses. | 1 | 2 | 3 | 4 | 5 |
| 63. Your organization's financial status. | 1 | 2 | 3 | 4 | 5 |
| 64. Your work group and departmental goals and objectives for this year. | 1 | 2 | 3 | 4 | 5 |
| 65. Your organization's strategic plans for the next few years. | 1 | 2 | 3 | 4 | 5 |
| 66. Results of clients' satisfaction surveys. | 1 | 2 | 3 | 4 | 5 |
| 67. Professionals' satisfaction with their multidisciplinary collaboration. | 1 | 2 | 3 | 4 | 5 |
| 68. Turnover and vacancy rate of professionals within your discipline in the organization. | 1 | 2 | 3 | 4 | 5 |
| 69. Colleagues' (within your discipline) satisfaction with their general practice. | 1 | 2 | 3 | 4 | 5 |
| 70. Colleagues' (within your discipline) satisfaction with their salaries and benefits. | 1 | 2 | 3 | 4 | 5 |
| 71. Management's opinion of the professional practice provided by your discipline. | 1 | 2 | 3 | 4 | 5 |
| 72. Other professional disciplines' opinion of the professional practice provided by your discipline. | 1 | 2 | 3 | 4 | 5 |
| 73. Your peers' opinion of their professional practice. | 1 | 2 | 3 | 4 | 5 |
| 74. Access to resources concerning recent advances in your practice (e.g. library, online). | 1 | 2 | 3 | 4 | 5 |

*In your hospital, please circle the group that has the ABILITY to:*

1 = Management/administration only
2 = Primarily management/administration with some staff input
3 = Equally shared by staff and management/administration
4 = Primarily staff with some management/administration input
5 = Staff only

## PART VI

| | 1 | 2 | 3 | 4 | 5 |
|---|---|---|---|---|---|
| 75. Negotiate solutions to conflicts among your professional colleagues. | 1 | 2 | 3 | 4 | 5 |
| 76. Negotiate solutions to conflicts between your professional colleagues and other professional groups. | 1 | 2 | 3 | 4 | 5 |
| 77. Negotiate solutions to conflicts between your professional colleagues and other organizational departments. | 1 | 2 | 3 | 4 | 5 |
| 78. Negotiate solutions to conflicts between your professional colleagues and their immediate managers. | 1 | 2 | 3 | 4 | 5 |
| 79. Negotiate solutions to conflicts between your professional colleagues and the organization's administration. | 1 | 2 | 3 | 4 | 5 |
| 80. Create a formal grievance procedure. | 1 | 2 | 3 | 4 | 5 |
| 81. Write the goals and objectives for your immediate work group. | 1 | 2 | 3 | 4 | 5 |
| 82. Write the philosophy, goals, and objectives of your department. | 1 | 2 | 3 | 4 | 5 |
| 83. Formulate the mission, philosophy, goals, and objectives of the organization. | 1 | 2 | 3 | 4 | 5 |
| 84. Write policies and procedures for your work group. | 1 | 2 | 3 | 4 | 5 |
| 85. Determine departmental policies and procedures. | 1 | 2 | 3 | 4 | 5 |
| 86. Determine organization-wide policies and procedures. | 1 | 2 | 3 | 4 | 5 |

## Shared Governance: A Practical Approach to Reshaping Professional Nursing Practice

### Target audience

Senior nurse executives and other members of organizational leadership

Nurse directors

Nurse managers

Nurse educators

Staff nurses

ANCC Magnet Recognition Program® coordinators/project directors

### Statement of Need:

This book identifies the essential elements of shared governance and provides practical strategies, case studies, best practices, and tips for leaders to design, implement, and assess shared governance process models in their facilities. (This activity is intended for individual use only.)

## Educational Objectives:

Upon completion of this activity, participants should be able to

1. Define the four primary principles of shared governance: partnership, equity, accountability, and ownership

2. Compare two professional nursing practice models

3. Describe the role of relational partnerships in shared governance

4. Describe four elements that are essential to the successful implementation of shared governance in the earliest stages of process development

5. Discuss the basic guidelines for forming the governance bodies in shared governance

6. Compare and contrast four structural process models of shared governance

7. Identify four strategic changes related to implementation of shared governance

8. Outline the three brain barriers to viable change in healthy organizations and the keys to overcome them

9. Describe the roles and responsibilities of a design team for implementation of shared governance

10. Discuss the purpose of bylaws and articles and how they are established when formalizing the shared governance structure

11. Discuss the roles of the following four stakeholders in shared governance: leadership, union representatives, community members, and patients

12. Discuss nursing's role in organization-wide shared governance related to the process structure or model, other disciplines and departments, and corporate and organizational integration

13. Describe how shared governance can be an integrating structure in healthcare organizations under nursing's leadership

14. Discuss the research project that looked at shared governance in a government agency using the Index of Professional Nursing Governance (IPNG)

15. Describe the six dimensions measured by the IPNG

16. Compare the attributes of a shared governance process model in organizations of different sizes and settings

17. Identify the two central elements of the Magnet Recognition Program® and the shared governance process

18. List the eight essentials of "magnetism" and how they compare to the shared governance process model

19. Describe at least ten tips for success when implementing shared governance

## Faculty

**Diana Swihart, PhD, DMin, MSN, CS, APRN,BC,** a clinical nurse specialist in nursing education at the Bay Pines (FL) VA Healthcare System, has a diverse background that includes many professional nursing arenas, theology, ministry, ancient Near Eastern studies, and archaeology.

**Katherine Riley, BSN, RN, CNA,BC** is an ANCC Magnet Recognition Program® (MRP) coordinator and assistant vice president of operations at Southwestern Vermont Medical Center in Bennington.

**Polly H. Willis, MSN, RN** is the MRP coordinator and the director of Saint Joseph's Stroke Center at Saint Joseph's Hospital, Atlanta.

## Accreditation/Designation Statement:

This educational activity for three (3) nursing contact hours is provided by HCPro, Inc. HCPro is accredited as a provider of continuing nursing education by the American Nurses Credentialing Center Commission on Accreditation.

## Disclosure Statements

HCPro, Inc. has a conflict of interest policy that requires course faculty to disclose any real or apparent commercial financial affiliations related to the content of their presentations/ materials. It is not assumed that these financial interests or affiliations will have an adverse impact on faculty presentations; they are simply noted here to fully inform the participants.

## Instructions

In order to be eligible to receive your nursing contact hours for this activity, you are required to do the following:

1. Read the book, *Shared Governance: A Practical Approach to Reshaping Professional Nursing Practice*
2. Complete the exam
3. Complete the evaluation
4. Provide your contact information on the exam and evaluation
5. Submit exam and evaluation to HCPro, Inc.

Please provide all of the information requested above and mail or fax your completed exam, program evaluation, and contact information to

> HCPro, Inc.
> Attention: Continuing Education Department
> 200 Hoods Lane
> P.O. Box 1168
> Marblehead, MA 01945
> Fax: 781/639-0179

**NOTE:**

This book and associated exam are intended for individual use only. If you would like to provide this continuing education exam to other members of your nursing staff, please contact our customer service department at 877/727-1728 to place your order. The exam fee schedule is as follows:

| Exam Quantity | Fee |
| --- | --- |
| 1 | $0 |
| 2–25 | $15 per person |
| 26–50 | $12 per person |
| 51–100 | $8 per person |
| 101+ | $5 per person |

## Continuing Education Exam

Name: _____

Title: _____

Facility Name: _____

Address: _____

City: _____ State: _____ Zip: _____

Phone Number: _____ Fax Number: _____

E-mail: _____

Date Completed: _____

1.  The best method for integrating staff roles and relationships into structures and processes to achieve positive patient outcomes is
    a. partnership.
    b. equity.
    c. accountability.
    d. ownership.

2.  Which of the following models embraces a philosophical foundation and operational framework for providing nursing services through relationships in an environment that embodies the concepts of partnership, equity, accountability, and ownership in shared governance?
    a. The Relationship-Based Care Model
    b. The Team Nursing Model
    c. The Case Management Model
    d. The Hierarchical Model

3.  In moving from hierarchy to relational partnerships in shared governance, the staff nurse moves from the _____ in the organization.
    a. center to the bottom
    b. bottom to the center
    c. center to the top
    d. top to the center

4. **Who must be invested in process empowerment and willing to undertake the efforts and energy necessary to implement shared governance?**
    a. Patients
    b. Physicians
    c. Staff nurses
    d. Committed nurse executives

5. **When forming the governance bodies, decisional groups must be**
    a. responsibility based.
    b. authority based.
    c. accountability based.
    d. larger than 20 members.

6. **Which of the following models follows traditional organizational lines of management and practice with each having separate groups that address specific functions and accountabilities?**
    a. Congressional model of shared governance
    b. Councilor model of shared governance
    c. Administrative model of shared governance
    d. Unit-based model of shared governance

7. **Strategic individual changes related to implementation of shared governance include**
    a. honesty and integrity.
    b. career enhancement programs.
    c. salaried work roles.
    d. increasing dependence on interdependence.

8. **The scenario in which people resist transitioning from doing the wrong thing well, to doing the right, new thing poorly, is called failure to**
    a. see.
    b. move.
    c. finish.
    d. reward.

9. Building an information base to understand and structure the work involved in implementing shared governance is one of the first responsibilities of the design team as members

  a. learn about shared governance and how it works.

  b. select a shared governance process structure or model.

  c. identify tasks and create a timeline.

  d. evaluate goals and process outcomes.

10. Which category of articles is identified through a credentialing and privileging mechanism?

  a. Roles in the organizational system

  b. Services provided by the organization

  c. Membership

  d. Governance structure

11. Obtaining affiliations with local universities and colleges for nurses to continue their academic education on hospital grounds is an example of a task performed by which of following stakeholders in shared governance?

  a. Leadership

  b. Union

  c. Community

  d. Patients

12. All disciplines and departments that have some role in making decisions that affect the direction and the operation of the organization is called a(n)

  a. integrating structure.

  b. universal process model.

  c. corporate integration.

  d. institutional process model.

13. Shared governance is an integrating structure that partners the

  a. manager with the staff nurse.

  b. patient with the physician.

  c. physician with the staff nurse.

  d. staff nurse with the patient.

14. **IPNG is an acronym for the**
    a. Institute of Professional Nursing Governance.
    b. Index of Professional Nursing Governance.
    c. Institute of Personal Nursing Governance.
    d. Index of Personal Nursing Governance.

15. **Which of the following is a subscale of the "resources" dimension used to measure nurses' perceptions of professional nursing governance facility-wide at the Durham (NC) VA Medical Center?**
    a. Interdisciplinary team members
    b. Evidence-based practice
    c. Unit budgets and expenditures
    d. Monitoring and securing supplies

16. **Despite their differences in size and setting, both a 410-bed tertiary care hospital and a 99-bed rural community hospital have found that shared governance requires _____ to sustain its effectiveness.**
    a. patience
    b. funding
    c. evolution
    d. consultation

17. **The two elements that are central to the Magnet Recognition Program® and the shared governance process are:**
    a. Cultural and hierarchal enhancements
    b. Achievement and responsibility enhancements
    c. Cultural and structural enhancements
    d. Structural and achievement enhancements

18. The following statement describes which of the eight essentials of "magnetism" list- ed below? "Doing what is needed for the staff first so they can focus all their energy, expertise, and experience on meeting the needs of the patients..."

    a. Adequate nurse staffing

    b. Control over nursing practice and environment

    c. Working with clinically competent nurses

    d. Concern for the patient is paramount

19. To which Force of Magnetism does this excerpt apply? "Staff nurses are involved in the decision making about budgets, schedules, salaries, competencies, resources, and practice. Creative and flexible staffing models and schedules accommodate the many demands staff nurses experience on their time and attention at work and at home."

    a. Force 1: Quality of nursing leadership

    b. Force 4: Personnel policies and programs

    c. Force 9: Autonomy

    d. Force 12: Image of nursing

20. One tip for successfully implementing shared governance is to communicate the process, expectations, roles, and _____ for nurses engaged in shared decision making throughout the organization, not just on the units.

    a. responsibilities

    b. behaviors

    c. attitudes

    d. salaries

## Continuing Education Evaluation

Name: _____

Title: _____

Facility Name: _____

Address: _____

City: _____ State: _____ Zip: _____

Phone Number: _____ Fax Number: _____

E-mail: _____

Date Completed: _____


1.   **This activity met the learning objectives stated:**
   • Define the four primary principles of shared governance: partnership, equity, accountability, and ownership

       Strongly Agree        Agree        Disagree        Strongly Disagree

   • Compare two professional nursing practice models

       Strongly Agree        Agree        Disagree        Strongly Disagree

   • Describe the role of relational partnerships in shared governance

       Strongly Agree        Agree        Disagree        Strongly Disagree

   • Describe four elements that are essential to the successful implementation of shared governance in the earliest stages of process development

       Strongly Agree        Agree        Disagree        Strongly Disagree

   • Discuss the basic guidelines for forming the governance bodies in shared governance

       Strongly Agree        Agree        Disagree        Strongly Disagree

   • Compare and contrast four structural process models of shared governance

       Strongly Agree        Agree        Disagree        Strongly Disagree

- Identify four strategic changes related to implementation of shared governance

  Strongly Agree        Agree        Disagree        Strongly Disagree

- Outline the three brain barriers to viable change in healthy organizations and the keys to overcome them

  Strongly Agree        Agree        Disagree        Strongly Disagree

- Describe the roles and responsibilities of a design team for implementation of shared governance

  Strongly Agree        Agree        Disagree        Strongly Disagree

- Discuss the purpose of bylaws and articles and how they are established when formalizing the shared governance structure

  Strongly Agree        Agree        Disagree        Strongly Disagree

- Discuss the roles of the following four stakeholders in shared governance: leadership, union representatives, community members, and patients

  Strongly Agree        Agree        Disagree        Strongly Disagree

- Discuss nursing's role in organization-wide shared governance related to the process structure or model, other disciplines and departments, and corporate and organizational integration

  Strongly Agree        Agree        Disagree        Strongly Disagree

- Describe how shared governance can be an integrating structure in healthcare organizations under nursing's leadership

  Strongly Agree        Agree        Disagree        Strongly Disagree

- Discuss the research project that looked at shared governance in a government agency using the Index of Professional Nursing Governance (IPNG)

  Strongly Agree        Agree        Disagree        Strongly Disagree

- Describe the six dimensions measured by the IPNG

  Strongly Agree          Agree          Disagree          Strongly Disagree

- Compare the attributes of a shared governance process model in organizations of different sizes and settings

  Strongly Agree          Agree          Disagree          Strongly Disagree

- Identify the two central elements of the ANCC Magnet Recognition Program® and the shared governance process

  Strongly Agree          Agree          Disagree          Strongly Disagree

- List the "eight essentials of magnetism" and how they compare to the shared governance process model

  Strongly Agree          Agree          Disagree          Strongly Disagree

- Describe at least ten tips for success when implementing shared governance

  Strongly Agree          Agree          Disagree          Strongly Disagree

2.  **Objectives were related to the overall purpose/goal of the activity:**

  Strongly Agree          Agree          Disagree          Strongly Disagree

3.  **This activity was related to my continuing education needs:**

  Strongly Agree          Agree          Disagree          Strongly Disagree

4.  **The exam for the activity was an accurate test of the knowledge gained:**

  Strongly Agree          Agree          Disagree          Strongly Disagree

5.  **The activity avoided commercial bias or influence:**

  Strongly Agree          Agree          Disagree          Strongly Disagree

6.  **This activity met my expectations:**

  Strongly Agree          Agree          Disagree          Strongly Disagree

7. **Will this activity enhance your professional practice?**
   Yes          No

8. **The format was an appropriate method for delivery of the content for this activity:**
   Strongly Agree          Agree          Disagree          Strongly Disagree

9. **If you have any comments on this activity please note them here:**

10. **How much time did it take for you to complete this activity?**

Thank you for completing this evaluation of our continuing education activity!

**Return completed form to:**
HCPro, Inc. • Attention: Continuing Education Department • 200 Hoods Lane, Marblehead, MA 01945
Telephone: 877/727-1728 • Fax: 781/639-2982